Chakra

for everyday living

D0063715

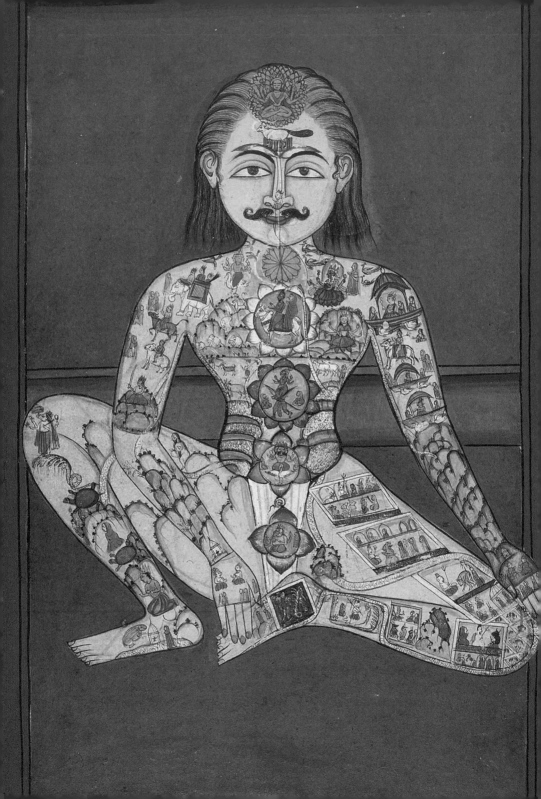

Chakra
for everyday living

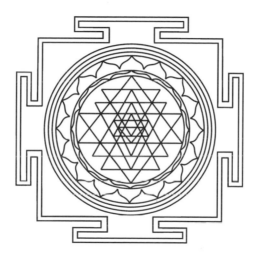

Liz Simpson and Patricia Mercier

An Hachette UK Company
www.hachette.co.uk

This edition published in 2015 by Bounty Books,
a division of Octopus Publishing Group Ltd
Carmelite House
50 Victoria Embankment
London, EC4Y 0DZ
www.octopusbooks.co.uk

ISBN: 978-0-7537-2975-5

A CIP catalogue record for this book is available
from the British Library

Printed and bound in China

10 9 8 7 6 5 4 3 2

CONTENTS

A LIFE IN BALANCE

The word *chakra* comes from the Sanskrit, meaning 'wheel' or 'disk'. These moderators of subtle energy are traditionally depicted as lotus flowers, each one resonating at a different frequency, corresponding to the one of the colours of the rainbow.

SEVEN MAJOR CHAKRAS

Although the human energy system is said to have many chakras, and new ones are being 'discovered' all the time, the traditional Hindu system names seven major ones. These are positioned with the stems of each lotus flower metaphysically 'embedded' into the spinal column, or *sushumna*, from the coccyx to the crown of the head.

THE RIGHT BALANCE

The chakra system offers a valuable explanation of the holistic nature of humankind. It outlines how, in order to maintain a healthy, balanced life, we must attend not just to certain physical dysfunctions that may occur but to our emotional, intellectual, and spiritual needs as well. Each of the seven chakras deals with different parts of this bigger picture and directs us to those areas where we might be functioning out of balance.

HUMAN ENERGY FIELDS

As a different consciousness dawns at the beginning of a new millennium we are at last shaking off the confines of a purely scientific approach to life and embracing concepts that were accepted by our ancestors many thousands of years ago. Interestingly, many scientists who have become disillusioned with mainstream explanations – and the arrogance of an orthodoxy that, when it can't explain a phenomenon, dismisses it as fanciful or non-existent – are using scientific methods to explain and prove many of life's anomalies. We explore some of these new advances in the following pages, where we look at how the human 'aura', depicted in ancient drawings as sheaths of white or golden light surrounding the bodies of saints or mystics, is simply a vibrational form of energy that – until recently – could not be recorded on scientific instruments. Our ancestors, more open-minded to things they could not see, let alone explain, had no need of such technology, since we are already equipped with an inbuilt sensor for this electromagnetic energy – our hands. As we journey together through the chakras we need only to prepare ourselves similarly – principally with an open mind. What we once took for granted as solid matter, thought to be made up of 'billiard ball' atoms, is – according to quantum physicists - simply 99.9999% empty space filled with energy. The fact that we cannot physically detect our chakras or aura can be explained thus: they operate as energy fields vibrating at a rate normally undetectable by the human eye and brain. As we take this journey together, and appreciate the very real benefits that come from balancing our human energy system, we will learn to discard the need for material evidence of their existence, since personal experience and enhanced well-being will provide this for us.

THE HOLISTIC VIEW

The origins of the sevenfold chakra system we shall be working through is buried in the roots of Hindu culture. The earliest mention of the term 'chakra' is said to come from the Vedas, the four holy books of the Hindus believed to date back before 2,500 BC, in which the god Vishnu is described as descending to Earth carrying in his four arms a chakra, a lotus flower, a club, and a conch

shell. However since the time of pre-Vedic societies, in which mystics and yogis passed down their knowledge through the spoken, rather than written, word, the notion of seven 'maps of consciousness' for optimum well-being goes back much further.

But why should we want to utilize a system that is rooted so far back in time? What relevance does it have to living in this day and age? In common with so many ancient practices, the chakra system takes a complete view of human experience. It integrates the natural tendency for equilibrium into the many layers that make up the self – the physical, mental, emotional, and spiritual. Chakra healing is based on the belief that in order for total well-being to take place we must act as an integrated whole.

In the first chapter we learn that the chakras operate like interconnected, self-opening, valves that channel the 'electrical current' of the Universal Life Force into the body. When there is a dysfunction or blockage in one part of the system it has an impact on all the other parts. Such malfunctioning can occur when the energy flowing through the chakras is either excessive or deficient. This book will help you recognize how such blockages, or dysfunctions, relate to any problems you may be experiencing and how, by using any or all of the techniques outlined in the following chapters, you can transform all aspects of your life for the better.

PART I

CHAKRA WELL-BEING

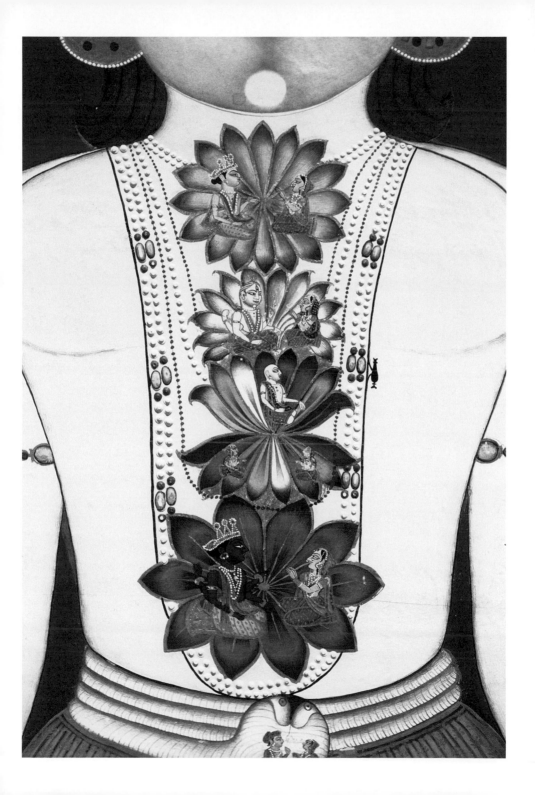

THE SPIRIT OF ENERGY

While anatomically undetectable, the seven major chakras are metaphysically linked with a number of different systems within the physical body. In this section we explore how the chakras bridge the visible, physical, self – in the form of the spinal cord, the autonomic nervous system, and the endocrine system – with our 'subtle' body, that envelope of vibrational energy that surrounds us, called the 'aura'.

While orthodox medicine describes our physical system in terms of chemistry, what is now understood is that for any chemical action to take place a change in the electromagnetic energy of the body must occur. This energy emanates from the 'mind' and explains the importance of the mind-body link to our physical, emotional, and mental health. The old scientific paradigm of relating to health purely in terms of the 'visible' is now being superseded by an appreciation of 'truths' once embraced only by mystics: that thoughts and the mind precede and affect physical matter. After all, what is thought but a form of energy?

THE ENDOCRINE SYSTEM

This system is one of the body's main physical control mechanisms. It comprises a number of ductless glands that are responsible for the production of many different natural chemicals called hormones. These chemical messengers, which include adrenalin, insulin, oestrogen, and progesterone, are secreted into the bloodstream from specific organs in the body to stimulate or inhibit certain physical processes.

The endocrine system, along with the autonomic nervous system, helps maintain the parameters needed for optimum health by adjusting levels of hormone secretion to suit special demands. In the same way that an imbalance in one chakra affects all of the other chakras, the nervous and endocrine systems are functionally interconnected andit follows that any disturbance in one part can lead to a malfunction elsewhere.

For a better understanding of how the endocrine system links with the chakras, we shall look at each pair in turn on the following pages.

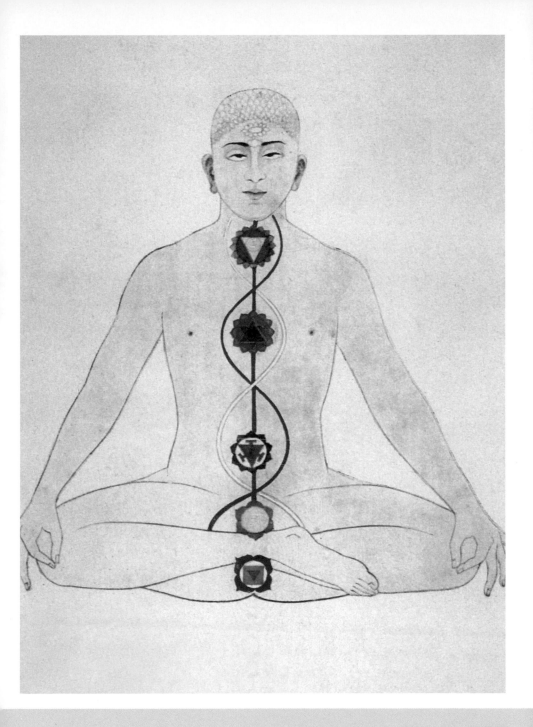

1 The Root Chakra and the adrenal glands

The adrenal glands are small, triangular-shaped glands that cap each of the two kidneys. These glands secrete a variety of hormones, including those that regulate the body's metabolism of fats, proteins and carbohydrates, and ones that control the balance of salt in our bodily fluids. These glands also produce adrenalin, a hormone that is considered essential for our primitive 'fight or flight' response. It is from this hormone that we can determine the link between this gland and the Root Chakra's association with the issue of physical survival.

2 The Sacral Chakra and the ovaries/testes

The male and female reproductive organs, or gonads, produce hormones that are responsible for the development of secondary sexual characteristics, such as the depth of voice we have or the amount of body hair. The testes and ovaries also control an individual's sexual development and maturity as well as the production of sperm in males and eggs in females. Our personal relationship with our own sexuality, and issues of emotional balance concerning that, is a key association of this chakra.

3 The Solar Plexus Chakra and the pancreas

The pancreas lies behind the stomach and secretes a variety of substances essential for the effective digestion of food. It also produces insulin, which helps control the blood's sugar level. One of the physical dysfunctions of this chakra is diabetes, a disease caused by excess sugar in the bloodstream. There is a further link with the Solar Plexus and adrenalin, which is why we experience 'butterflies in the stomach' during frightening experiences. The associated body parts the digestive system and a further dysfunction of this chakra is stomach ulcers.

4 The Heart Chakra and the thymus gland

Located just above the heart, the thymus produces hormones that stimulate general growth, particularly early in life. It also has a purifying role in the body by stimulating the production of lymphocytes, which form part of the blood's white cells' defence system, attacking invading organisms and providing immunity. Scientists now recognize that autoimmune diseases, where the immune system attacks its own proteins, mistaking them for a foreign substance, have an emotional link and are not simply due to physical or environmental causes.

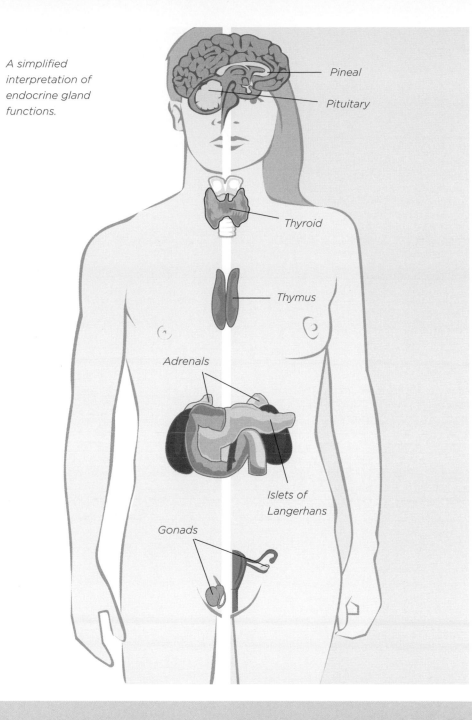

A simplified interpretation of endocrine gland functions.

Pineal

Pituitary

Thyroid

Thymus

Adrenals

Islets of Langerhans

Gonads

5 The Throat Chakra and the thyroid/parathyroid glands

The thyroid gland is situated on either side of the larynx and trachea in the neck. It manufactures thyroxine, which controls the body's metabolic rate - that is, how effectively the body converts food into energy. Behind the thyroid gland lies the parathyroid gland, which controls the level of calcium in the bloodstream.

In addition to physical growth, these glands are also believed to affect one's mental development. The Throat Chakra, linked with all forms of communication, corresponds to the need for balance between the rational, cerebral, approach and the emotional expression of the heart.

6 The Brow Chakra and the pituitary gland

The pituitary gland is located within a structure at the base of the skull, close to the eyebrows. It was once called the 'master gland' of the endocrine system, and has since been found to be controlled by hormonal substances released by the hypothalmus, a part of the brain. This vital gland influences growth, metabolism, and general body chemistry. This includes the hormone that produces contractions during labour and releases milk from the breasts during lactation. It is interesting to note this Third Eye-pituitary gland connection with birth and motherhood, a time when many women feel that their intuition, particularly with regard to their child, is at its peak.

7 The Crown Chakra and the pineal gland

The glandular connection of the Crown Chakra is the pineal gland, a pea-sized body that lies deep within the brain and was once thought to serve no useful purpose.

Considered in the seventeenth century to be the seat of the soul by French philosopher, René Descartes, recent scientific research has linked this gland with the production of melatonin and regulates our internal 'body clock'. Melatonin is also the subject of intense scientific interest for its possible anti-ageing properties and is believed to affect the pituitary, thyroid, adrenals, and gonads - although no one yet understands how or why. Like the Crown's function within the chakra system as a whole, the pineal gland is considered the control centre for the effective functioning of our physical, emotional, and mental selves.

THE SUSHUMNA AND KUNDALINI RISING

In the same way that our physical body's central nervous system consists of the spinal cord leading to the brain, the energetic equivalent – the *sushumna* – is the vertical column within which the seven chakras are located. The parallels between these physical and metaphysical structures are striking.

UNIVERSAL LIFE FORCE

Whereas the function of the spinal cord is to relay impulses to and from the brain and other parts of the body, the *sushumna* channels energy from the Universal Life Force to and from the Crown and Root Chakras. Each chakra is rooted into the *sushumna* by both a front and a rear aspect.

In their traditional depictions as lotus flowers, the petals of each chakra emerge from the *sushumna* at the front of the body, while the stems open out from the back. The stems normally remain closed and have a negative polarity, whereas the petals consecutively vibrate, rotate in a clockwise or anticlockwise direction, as well as open and close. They have a positive polarity.

The journey upward through the chakras is spoken of in terms of 'Kundalini rising'. Kundalini is the serpent goddess, often depicted as coiled three and a half times around the Root Chakra. According to Hindu tradition, when awakened Kundalini pierces each chakra in turn as she travels from the root toward the crown. Once she has arrived at her destination the subject is said to have achieved enlightenment.

THE SERPENT IN RELIGION

There are many links between Kundalini and religious and cultural archetypes. In Genesis it is a serpent that leads Adam and Eve to taste from the Tree of Knowledge, thereby instigating the inner conflict between material needs and the spiritual desire to achieve higher states of consciousness. And in Egypt, the pharaohs wore serpent symbols over the Third Eye Chakra to represent godlike stature. It is the appreciation of our Higher Self - finding the God within - that is the ultimate goal of this journey through the chakras.

THE HUMAN AURA

The peoples of the ancient cultures of the East, who developed the notion of a sevenfold chakra system, knew and understood that beyond its material form the body is really a pulsating, dynamic field of energy.

The concept of an 'aura', depicted in early paintings as a halo of bright, multi-coloured light around the physical self, defies the laws of physics but only as we currently understand them. Orthodox science may have been unable to measure this 'spiritual' energy - in the same way that it is incapable of measuring emotional or mental energy - but there is no denying these levels of experience exist.

Pioneering experts in the United States and China, however, now say that the bioelectromagnetic field – or aura – of every living thing is no longer in question. Using technology developed from the NASA space programme in the United States, for example, neurophysiologist and psychologist Dr Valerie V. Hunt has scientifically verified that there are two primary electrical systems in the physical body. The first is the alternating electrical current of the nervous system and brain which governs our muscles, hormones, and physical sensations. The second is a continuous, electromagnetic radiation coming off our atoms which allows for an energy exchange between individuals and their environment.

Each person's unique energy field - said to surround them like an envelope - is accessed from a universal pool known as the Universal Life Force, 'prana', or 'chi' (or Qi). This pool of energy is drawn into the body through each of the chakras and is transformed by them into a particular quality, dominant sense, and emotional correlate. The chakras act like a series of valves in a system connecting a water tap to a garden hose. Once the tap is turned on, the water should flow smoothly through the system. But if there is a kink in the hose (analogous to a blockage of energy) or if any of the valves are too open or too closed, this affects the proper functioning of the whole unit.

Experts now believe that the field of radiation, which we call the aura, in combination with our DNA, makes up our combined genetic material.

It seems that while the passive DNA preserves our unique genetic code, the transmitting bioelectromagnetic field is able to modify it. Ancient healers believed that the aura holds the key to a person's physical, mental, emotional, and spiritual states. Scientists working in the field of energy medicine back this up, saying that this vibrating energy field, banded in layers around the physical body like a set of Russian dolls, is similar to the magnetic tape of a tape recorder which stores coded information about our past, present, and future health. And that by maintaining an open and smooth flowing channel of energy through our chakras, by freeing ourselves of the mental or emotional traumas that can cause blockages, we can pre-empt the onset of physical 'dis-ease'. See the following pages for ways in which you can use the information in the rest of this book to re-balance your own chakra system.

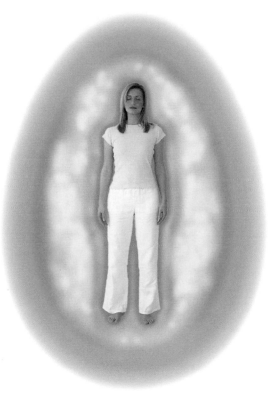

A smooth, steady flow of energy through the chakra system ensures a healthy aura, in turn indicating a body clear from conflict.

CHAKRA BALANCING

As you read this book you will discover various ways to bring the chakras into balance, as you learn how meditation, aromatherapy, crystals, and yoga as well as other techniques are used.

UNDERSTANDING THE CONDITION OF THE CHAKRAS

To balance the chakras, you must first be clear about the condition that each individual chakra is in, and interpret this in terms of energy flow through these 'wheels of light'.

People who can see the luminous auric field perceive chakras as vortices of swirling lights, spiralling into contact with the physical body at key points corresponding to particular parts of the body, both front and back.

The exceptions are the Crown Chakra, which opens upwards above the head, and the Root Chakra, which opens downwards from the perineum. Some people describe the chakras as being either 'open' or 'closed', but there are better descriptions for the chakra qualities, as described on page 20.

WAYS TO BALANCE THE CHAKRAS

In the same way that no one alternative health approach suits everybody, and you may need to experience several before you discover the one that works best for you, there are various different ways of balancing your chakras. The following pages explain the various approaches outlined in the following chakra section of the book. Try them all; there is bound to be one that resonates with you and becomes your favourite. However, it is important to sample the others, too. Even if you feel pre-disposed to focusing on the yoga-based exercises, for example, there may be occasions when it is inconvenient to practise them for a few days. At such times it may be helpful to exercise your mind by reflecting on the archetypes linked with the chakras, doing some meditation or guided visualizations, or keeping a daily questions journal.

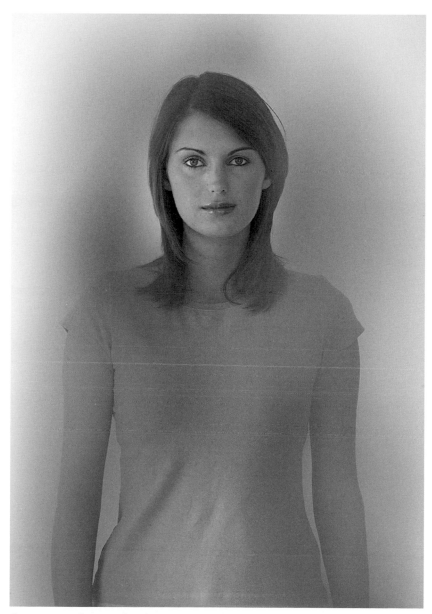

An aura may be seen by clairvoyants and by Kirlian photography.

CHAKRA QUALITIES

- **Active:** The chakra is functioning as intended, showing a healthy input and output of energy. The person in question will normally be fit and healthy. Different parts of their energy field – the emotional, mental and spiritual bodies – will all be vibrant as well.

- **Underactive:** The chakra in question needs some type of stimulation, perhaps in order to cope with adverse conditions in the physical body or in the energy field.

- **Passive/balanced:** The chakra energies are either 'at rest' or in a steady, harmonious balance of input and output.

- **Overactive:** The chakra is overstimulated, possibly because it is trying to eliminate imbalances in the physical body. Our luminous bodies can have undesirable energies. Overactivity of certain chakras may be due to them trying to eliminate long-held imprints that are detrimental to our well-being (such as the imprints of addiction or abuse).

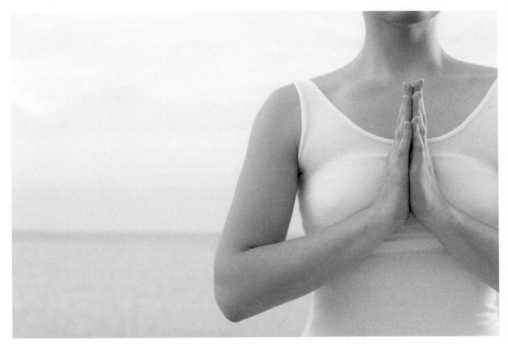

A relaxed body sends increased subtle energy through your whole chakra system.

ARCHETYPES

These are universal themes, or models, of the 'human condition'. Illustrated through myths, fairy stories, and even modern films, they provide us with an understanding of our emotional experiences – both what we are and what we would like to become. Through these 'life dramas' we learn about the different values that underpin our attitudes, beliefs and behaviours.

Archetypal storytelling polarizes the choices we make in tackling life's challenges; whether to opt for courage or cowardice, patience or impetuousness, thought or action. Archetypes are far more 'black and white' than real life is, so that we can see more clearly the choices on offer. However, there are times when both functional and dysfunctional archetypes are valuable for spiritual growth. While we may choose to suppress our 'dark side' we should accept that we can never totally eradicate it. Our mission toward self-ownership and enlightenment includes acknowledging those parts of ourselves that we may not instinctively like or admire; our free will is strengthened from never letting them have total power over us.

By identifying the patterns we may have embedded into our neural pathways and which are outwardly projected as particular behaviours, we can choose to discard those that no longer serve us. There are both dysfunctional and functional archetypes associated with each chakra. Understanding how these influence our lives can help us take up the reins of the emotional challenges that face us so that we can choose to take a different direction and move on to a new stage of development.

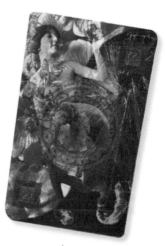

A depiction of the Root Chakra archetypes: The Earth Mother and the Victim.

MEDITATION

Psychologists have discovered that the brain cannot differentiate between what is real and what is realistically imagined. There are many benefits to be derived from taking part in regular meditations and guided visualizations.

In the Yoga Sutras of Patanjali (written advice for yoga practitioners), there are three stages for training the mind:

• **Concentration Dharana**, whose aim is to focus the inner experience.

• **Meditation Dhyana**, whose aim is to expand the inner experience.

• **Contemplation Samadhi**, whose aim is to deepen the inner experience.

DHARANA

The daily practice of concentration ideally comes after you have finished your yoga asanas. In the Raja system of yoga, which is regarded as one of the highest disciplines, it is usual to make specific times to practise it. Concentration of the mind might be on an abstract idea or an object. In concentration you try to avoid the chain association in your mind; for example, when you think of an orange, you may think of the tree – the sunshine that helped the tree grow – you wonder who picked the fruit. That is not dharana; in dharana you concentrate solely on the orange. The aim is to still the restless inner dialogue. Practicing at dawn can increase its effectiveness.

DHYANA

When dhyana is reached, it is no longer necessary to practise concentration, because at this point on your spiritual journey, daily meditation replaces concentration. The term 'meditation' can mean many things to many people. However, in the context of Patanjali's system and Raja yoga, dhyana means the following: whereas dharana contracts the mind, dhyana expands the mind around the subject. You enlarge the field of consciousness to take in the spiritual nature of (in this simple example) an orange. For most people, dhyana/contemplation is the final stage – samadhi is rarely reached.

SAMADHI

Of course, the practice of meditation does not normally use objects like an orange! To reach samadhi you are more likely to work with an abstract concept, such as unconditional love or a line from a sacred text.

Samadhi may be interpreted as uniting the lower consciousness or self with super-consciousness or the higher self. The highest principle, as Patanjali said, 'is when the mind is so far concerned with the object alone, to a degree of one's seeming non-existence, that is Samadhi'.

However, not all meditation necessarily ends in the blissful state of samadhi. Experienced meditators say that samadhi comes when you least expect it, and you should not try to analyse the journey.

'Without leaving his house, one can know everything that is necessary. Without leaving himself one can grasp all wisdom.'

-Lao Tzu

YANTRAS

The yantras are intricate symbols that are used to represent each chakra and can be a useful meditation tool. They are the yogi equivalent of the Buddhist mandala: visual symbols of complex spiritual concepts. Each chakra yantra is based on a lotus, the traditional symbol of enlightenment in Hindu and Buddhist thought.

The increasing number of lotus petals in each chakra, as we ascend the ladder, suggests the rising energy or vibrational frequencies of the respective chakras – each functioning as a transformer of energies from one potency to another. The yantra for each chakra also contains specific symbols relevant to that chakra. We will explore these in greater detail in the sections devoted to the chakras.

HOW TO USE YANTRAS

If you are using yantras in meditation, place them so that you can see them on the level and can focus upon them comfortably. Traditionally a yantra is considered to be more powerful than a picture of a god, which, to be energized, requires a yantra to be affixed at its base or back and used together with a mantra. It is generally recommended that a drawing or print of a yantra is placed in the north/north-west direction of a room, facing the south/south-east direction. However, the special Sri Yantra, considered to be the 'mother' form of all yantras, is traditionally placed in the east, facing west.

THE YANTRAS AS A CENTRING DEVICE

Yantras are powerful 'centring' devices for harnessing divine energies. Centring means that you draw all your inner and outer focus to a still point at the centre of your mind. If you are centred, you will not be disturbed by events in your everyday life. Centring comes into its own when you use it as a preliminary focus before meditation.

It is said that our mind is like a troupe of monkeys leaping from branch to branch, feeding on the tastiest fruits and chattering all the time. Our task is to stop them leaping about, find a stillness and satisfaction in deep silence, and bring our attention to a fixed point. This could be an external object, such as a yantra, a candle flame or an inner perception (such as turning our closed eyes upwards towards the Brow Chakra). To gain the skill of centring, constantly but gently draw your awareness away from disturbing thoughts and towards the centre of your focus.

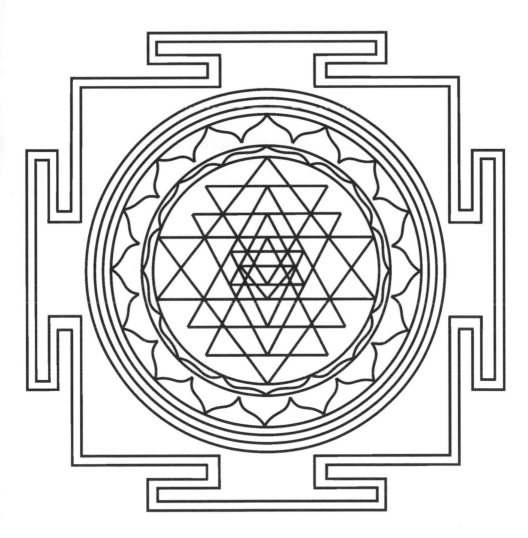

Yogis practise Tratakam (concentration, without eyes blinking) on the Sri Yantra.

AFFIRMATIONS

Every time you have a particular thought a neural pathway is created in the brain – a weak link at first, but one which gets stronger the more times the same thought is brought to mind.

That is why it is so difficult to break habitual patterns of thinking; they have become so embedded in our brain that we need to create another, more compelling, 'pathway' to compete with them. This is what we do when we say affirmations. These are positive sentences which 'tell' our brain that we are choosing to think differently about a particular life challenge. And just like the grass analogy, the more we speak and think these beneficial, optimistic messages to ourselves – the greater our chances of changing old, inappropriate, patterns of thought and behaviour.

DAILY QUESTIONS

The more we understand ourselves the better equipped we are to make positive changes in our lives. The questions that relate to each chakra's life challenge will help you unpick the ways in which you sabotage your happiness and well-being with dysfunctional behaviours. They will also help you determine how to bring about those physical, mental, emotional, and spiritual changes which will aid the more effective functioning of your chakras.

Keeping a journal is vital for self-development. We have so many thoughts each day it is difficult to keep pace with them and virtually impossible – unless we write them down – to ascertain the patterns that underpin our attitudes to life. As you make your journey through the chakras your journal will help you chart progress and motivate you toward personal development.

Write your thoughts nightly for the next three weeks. That's the length of time we need to perform a new behaviour in order to turn it into a habit. Don't worry about how much or how little you write. The important thing is to select a question that resonates with you and the particular challenge you are facing at this time, and let your consciousness lead you to the answer.

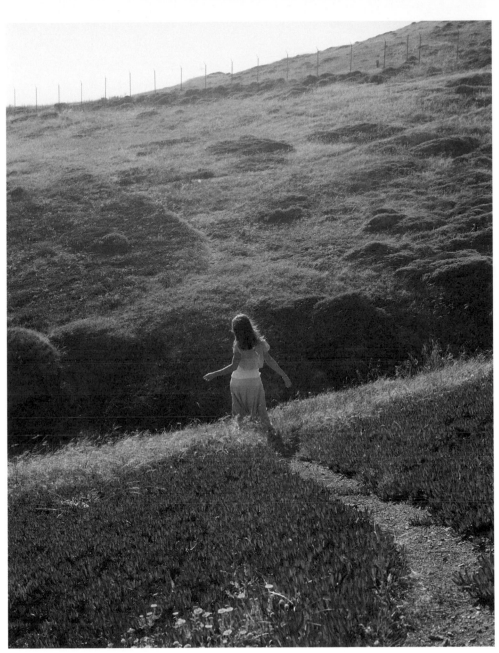

Like a well-trodden path, affirmations help to keep positive thoughts at the surface of our minds.

AROMATHERAPY

Aromatherapy is the use of volatile liquid plant materials (known as essential oils) and other aromatic plant compounds to enhance mood and health. Massage techniques using essential oils can benefit the chakras by clearing them of unwanted energies and rebalancing them.

CHAKRA MASSAGE

If you are giving aromatherapy to another person, it is best to get some training. Auric and chakra massage are done to another person when they are fully clothed.

If you are treating yourself or a friend, establish which oils to use, then place a 5 ml teaspoon of base carrier oil into a saucer and add one or two drops of your chosen essential oil.

1 Put just one drop of your combined essential and carrier oil into the palms of your hands, then rub them together for a moment.

2 Working only within the auric field, and not on the actual body, slowly sweep the palms of your hands down the front and back of the recipient. Do this until you perceive a change in their energy levels.

3 Alternatively, concentrate on one chakra area in the auric field, allowing your hands to move in a relaxed way in a spiralling pattern. Normally chakras are cleared of unwanted energies by spiralling anticlockwise and are returned to balance by spiralling clockwise.

4 Always wash your hands in cool water after cleansing or healing another person, in order to remove unwanted energies from your own auric field.

Caution: Never take essential oils orally. For massage on the skin always dilute them with base carrier oils. If your skin is sensitive, do a simple skin test first: make up the mix in the recommended dilution and apply a few drops to the inside crease of your elbow. Wait 24 hours to see if any irritant reaction occurs.

Note: During pregnancy, or for children under the age of 12, do not use essential oils (or ingest herbs) at all, except under the recommendation and supervision of a professional.

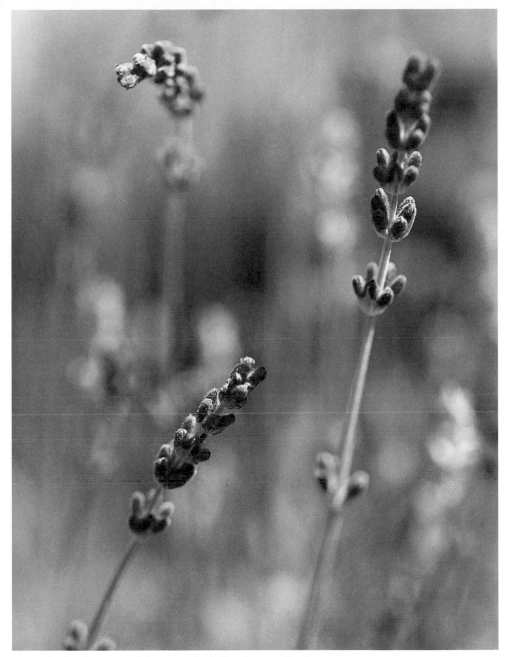

Lavender has been used therapeutically for thousands of years.

OILS FOR MASSAGE

Essential oils are extremely strong and are always mixed with a base or 'carrier' oil when used for massage. Always use high-quality extra-virgin cold-pressed oils as a base oil, and the best essential oils that you can buy from a specialist company.

Never use baby oil, since most types are made from a petro-chemical mineral oil that is not compatible with the skin. For massage on dry skin, use sweet almond oil with the addition of 10 per cent wheatgerm (check for nut and wheat allergies first) or avocado oil. The word 'natural' on a label is not sufficient: you need to be really sure you are getting 'pure essential oil'. Cheap oils sold for 'burners' or vaporizers must never be used on the skin.

When used in massage, essential oils are always diluted. For adults a general rule is 2.5 per cent essential oil to 97.5 per cent base oil. To ascertain this, measure your base oil in millilitres and divide by two; the answer gives the number of drops of essential oil that you should add – for example, 20 ml of base oil requires a maximum of ten drops.

OIL DIFFUSERS

You can combine essential oils' beautiful aromas with the power of heat and light by using an oil diffuser/ vaporizer. Put a little water into the reservoir, add up to five drops of neat essential oil and light a 'tea light' underneath. Place it in a safe place and, as the water evaporates, your room will be filled with a wonderful aroma. Alternatively, put a few drops of neat essential oil in a saucer of water on top of a radiator.

The aroma can be chosen to produce a relaxing, therapeutic, stimulating or sensual atmosphere. During illness an oil diffuser used with some of the more herbal-smelling oils – for example, sage, thyme, rosemary, tea tree or pine, in combination with lavender – can inhibit common airborne bacteria such as cold and influenza viruses. It may also help people who have difficulty breathing, but for severe conditions always take medical advice.

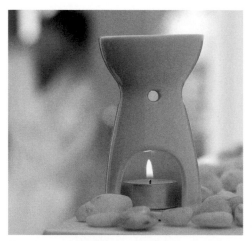

Burning oil in a diffuser can fill a room with wonderful aromas.

APPROPRIATE ESSENTIAL OILS FOR CHAKRA MASSAGE

Chakra	Qualities	Essential Oils
Root	Grounding/stabilizing Earth energy	Patchouli, myrrh, cedarwood
Sacral	Transmuting sexual energy	Sandalwood, jasmine, rose, ylang-ylang
Solar Plexus	Transducing solar and pranic energy	Sage, juniper, geranium
Heart	Flow of unconditional love	Rose, melissa, neroli
Throat	Self-expression, communication, will	Chamomile, lavender, rosemary, thyme
Brow	Balancing higher and lower selves, ESP	Frankincense, basil
Crown	Divine love and super-consciousness	Rosewood, ylang-ylang, linden

YOGA

Yoga is a branch of Indian philosophy that is concerned with the union of the individual together with the universal consciousness. Our knowledge of yoga is based on the Yoga Sutras, ancient Indian texts that describe the philosophy and practices of yoga.

They were written sometime during the period from the 5th century BCE to the 2nd century CE, and define an eight-limbed path (ashtanga) that must be followed in order to reach samadhi, where the spirit is liberated and joins the Universal Spirit.

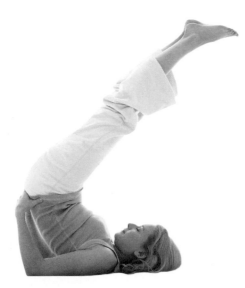

Yoga postures help to stretch and tone the body internally and externally.

TYPES OF HATHA YOGA

Ananda yoga: This style uses gentle postures designed to move the energy up to the brain and prepare the body for meditation. Classes also focus on proper body alignment and controlled breathing.

Ashtanga (or Astanga/Power) yoga: This form comprises a challenging series of poses that focus on strength and flexibility, by synchronizing movement with the breath.

Iyengar yoga: This focuses on body alignment. Practitioners hold each pose for a longer amount of time, and use props such as straps, blankets and wooden blocks.

Sivananda yoga: This traditional type of yoga concentrates on connecting the body to the Solar Plexus, where an enormous amount of energy is stored. A typical class will combine postures, breathing, dietary restrictions, chanting and meditation.

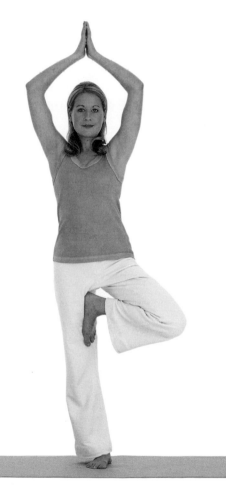

A yoga practitioner performing a simple 'tree' posture.

THE SIX MAIN YOGA PATHS

The term 'yoga' actually describes a number of different paths, not all of which are based on physical practices. The six main paths are:

- **Jnana yoga:** Where the practitioner pursues enlightenment via the path of knowledge, using study and meditation.

- **Bhakti yoga:** A path of devotion based on the worship of a god or guru.

- **Karma yoga:** A path to enlightenment based on selfless action.

- **Mantra yoga:** A path based on the repetition of sacred sound.

- **Raja yoga:** An eight-step path to enlightenment based on posture, breath control, meditation and the withdrawal of the senses.

- **Hatha yoga:** This is the type of yoga with which most people in the West are familiar – it is based on physical postures, breathing exercises, cleansing and mindful awareness.

HOW YOGA PRACTICE CAN HELP BALANCE THE CHAKRAS

Yoga practice is of specific benefit to the chakras because the postures (asanas) assist in freeing up prana. As you perform the bending, stretching and twisting poses, you help prana to flow freely throughout the energy channels, or nadi, of your body. Yoga is particularly helpful for the release of kundalini energy, helping it rise up through each chakra one by one, ascending up the spine to the crown. Kundalini energy can fail to rise if the bandhas, or body locks, are not in place. It also fails to rise if one or more of the chakras are blocked, but the regular practise of kundalini yoga can help to unblock the chakras.

The best way to practise yoga is by joining a reputable school and working progressively through each class. In this book we show the asanas that can be particularly beneficial for each chakra, but remember that it is important to warm up the body first, and always take medical advice if you have an existing health condition or have not performed physical exercise for some time.

Active asanas clear excess/negative energies from the whole body and auric field by ascending from Root to Crown. Passive asanas then draw prana into deep core level, harmonizing our energies as we descend back down the chakras from Crown to Root.

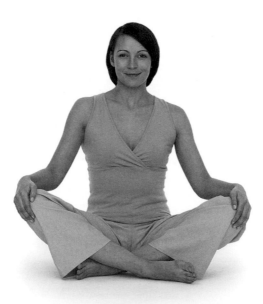

The lotus position, with the body seated motionless and at ease, in a cross-legged posture.

ACTIVE AND PASSIVE ASANAS FOR EACH CHAKRA

Active asanas

1 **Begin standing in balance:**
Pranamasana (prayer pose)

2 **Root Chakra:** Warrior

3 **Sacral Chakra:**
Twisting triangle

4 **Solar Plexus Chakra:**
Cow pose

5 **Heart Chakra:** Cobra pose

6 **Throat Chakra:** Bow pose

7 **Brow Chakra:**
Dog face-down pose

8 **Crown Chakra:** Headstand

Passive asanas

9 **Crown Chakra:**
Shoulder stand

10 **Brow Chakra:** Plough pose

11 **Throat Chakra:**
Sitting forward bend

12 **Heart Chakra:**
Head-to-knee pose

13 **Solar Plexus Chakra:**
Camel pose

14 **Sacral Chakra:** Pose of Shiva

15 **Base Chakra:** Eagle pose

16 **End sitting in balance:**
Lotus pose or simpler asana

For a full yoga session to balance every chakra, work through all the asanas from 1 to 16. Alternatively, refer to the relevant section of this book and select asanas for a specific chakra. However, you should always begin with a standing balance (1) and end with a sitting or balancing asana, such as the lotus (16). Instructions for each asana are given in the relevant chakra section. Asana positions are never forced – only stretch to your own comfortable level. If in doubt, join a yoga class or consult a qualified teacher.

Note: If you have a medical condition, do not attempt extreme asanas unless you have taken medical advice and are working under the direction of a qualified yoga teacher.

CRYSTALS

Healers observe that most 'dis-ease' is caused by an energy imbalance, usually a reduced flow of pranic life-force throughout the chakras. Crystals and gems help to realign, rebalance and energize the chakras into appropriate functions.

Our chakras have a sympathetic resonance with natural crystals, and researchers have now developed instruments that can measure an instantaneous fluctuation of electrical energy when a crystal (particularly quartz) comes near a chakra.

If you are unsure which crystals to use, you can always be effective with clear quartz, since it channels all the rainbow colours of the spectrum through its crystalline matrix. Learn to love the crystals you are using, and the inner Light within them will offer itself to you.

HOW TO CHOOSE CRYSTALS

Let your intuition guide you when you are collecting crystals, and try to have some idea as to what you want to do with them. For example, do you want them to look attractive in your room, change the energies in the home, or do you wish to use them for healing purposes?

Crystals do not have to be large or expensive to be effective. It is a good idea to get together a selection of crystal pebbles (tumbled stones) in the seven colours of the spectrum, together with two clear quartz 'points' about 5 cm (2 in) in length.

Ideally, keep your crystals wrapped in red silk when you are not using them, and cleanse their auric field before and after use.

HOW TO CLEANSE CRYSTALS

All hard crystals can safely be cleansed in clear water, or in water with a small pinch of salt in it. Then either put them into sunshine or moonlight to energize them. Other cleansing methods to try are: the smoke of incense, flower remedies, sound, meditation, Reiki healing or placing the crystal in the earth – ensure that each time you have love in your heart as you handle the crystals.

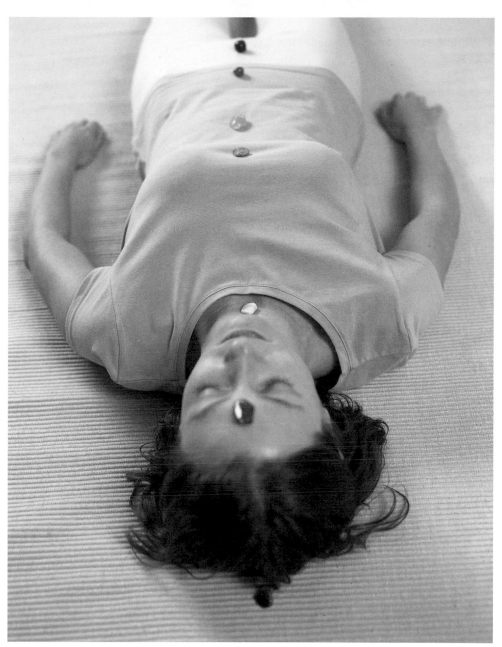

Relaxing and chakra balancing with crystal pebbles can help increase pranic life-force flow through the chakras.

HOW TO DEDICATE CRYSTALS

When a crystal first comes into your guardianship, hold it and get to know it, then cleanse and meditate with it. Then make a dedication. For example, you might say:

'May this crystal work only with the power of Unconditional Love and Light.'

or

'For the highest universal purpose of ...'

Here you can add 'clearing the auric field' or some other appropriate dedication.

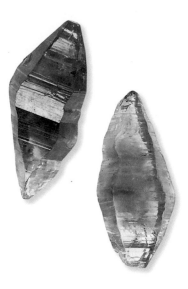

HOW TO USE CRYSTALS

After you have cleansed and dedicated a crystal, you are ready to use it in healing work, such as calming or balancing the chakras.

1 Hold it in your non-dominant hand close to the chakra in question, preferably against your skin, bringing it into contact with the body. Leave it there for some minutes.

2 Now move your hand away from your body by 5 cm (2 in). Wait some minutes.

3 Move your hand further away by 15 cm (6 in). Wait some minutes.

4 Move your hand 30 cm (12 in) away. Wait some minutes.

5 Move your hand an arm's length away from your body. Wait some minutes.

6 Each time you move your hand further away, imagine that you are linked to the crystal with a golden cord of light.

7 Finally move your hand and crystal in and out of your auric field over the chakra. You will find the position that feels most effective. Wait for some minutes, really 'connecting' to the crystal.

8 When you have finished, thank the crystal and cleanse it.

MAKING A CRYSTAL ESSENCE BY THE INDIRECT METHOD

You can add crystal essences to bath water, or slowly sip seven drops of the essence three times a day. The indirect method means that the crystal itself does not come into direct contact with water – only its vibration is transferred to the 'memory' of the water.

1 Clean any dust or dirt from your crystal with a soft feather. Cleanse the crystal psychically by intention, or with sound or incense.

2 Place the crystal in a clear glass jar, then stand the jar in a glass bowl of pure spring water. Put the bowl in sunlight for 12 hours to transfer the vibration of the crystal to the water. Alternatively, place a minimum of four large quartz crystal points around the outside of the bowl of water, pointing inwards.

3 If you wish to keep the essence for more than a few days, you need to preserve it in a solution of 50 per cent brandy/vodka to 50 per cent essence. All crystal essences should be kept in the cool and dark, away from strong smells, with the bottles not touching one another.

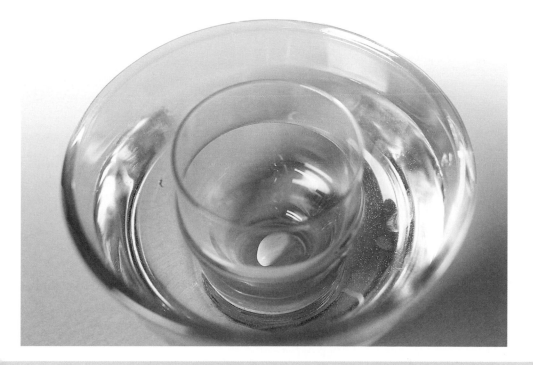

CHAKRA CORRESPONDENCES

Chakra Location	Sanskrit Name Meaning	Associated Colour	Main Issue
7 Crown Top of head	Sahasrara Thousandfold	Violet, gold, white	Spirituality
6 Brow Above and between eyebrows	Ajna To perceive, to know	Indigo	Intuition, wisdom
5 Throat Centrally, at base of neck	Vishuddha Purification	Blue	Communication, self-expression
4 Heart Centre of chest	Anahata Unstruck	Green, pink	Love and relationships
3 Solar Plexus Between navel and base of sternum	Manipura Lustrous gem	Yellow	Personal power, self will
2 Sacral Lower abdomen, between navel and genitals	Svadhisthana Sweetness	Orange	Emotional balance and sexuality
1 Root Between anus and genitals	Muladhara Root or support	Red	Survival and physical need

Glandular Connection	Associated Body Parts	Element Ruling Planet	Astrological Associations	Associated Sense
Pineal	Upper skull, cerebral cortex, skin	Thought, cosmic energy Uranus	Aquarius	Beyond Self
Pituitary	Eyes, base of skull	Light/ telepathic energy Jupiter	Saggitarius, Pisces	Sixth Sense
Thyroid, parathyroid	Mouth, throat, ears	Ether Mercury	Gemini, Virgo	Sound/hearing
Thymus	Heart and chest, lungs and circulation	Air Venus	Libra, Taurus	Touch
Pancreas	Digestive system, muscles	Fire Mars/Sun	Aries, Leo	Sight
Ovaries/Testes	Sex organs, bladder, prostate, womb	Water Pluto	Cancer, Scorpio	Taste
Adrenals	Bones, skeletal structure	Earth Saturn	Capricorn	Smell

CHAKRA CORRESPONDENCES

Chakra Location	Fragrances & Oils	Crystals	Animals Archtypes
7 Crown Top of the Head	Ylang-ylang, lime blossom, rosewood, lotus or waterlily	Celestite, blue sapphire, chaorite, sugilite, quartz, amethyst	(None) Guru/Egocentric
6 Brow Above and between eyebrows	Frankincense, basil	Diamond, emerald, sapphire, lapis lazuli	(None) Psychic/Rationalist
5 Throat Centrally, at base of neck	Lavender, rosemary, thyme, sage, chamomile	Blue topaz, yellow topaz, sapphire, emerald, quartz	Elephant, bull Communicator/ Masked Self
4 Heart Centre of chest	Rose, melissa, neroli	Peridot, pink topaz, pink or lavender kunzite, rhondite, watermelon tourmaline, rose quartz, rhodocrosite	Gazelle, antelope Lover/Performer
3 Solar Plexus Between navel and base of sternum	Clary sage, juniper, geranium	Topaz, yellow tourmaline, emerald, sapphire, citrine	Ram Spiritual warrior/ Drudge
2 Sacral Lower abdomen, between navel and genitals	Jasmine, rose, sandalwood	Fire opal, carnelian, emerald, moonstone, aquamarine	Fish-tailed alligator Sovereign/Martyr
1 Root Between anus and genitals	Cedarwood, patchouli, myrrh	Emerald, blue sapphire, carnelian	Elephant Earth Mother/Victim

Physical Dysfunctions	Emotional Dysfunctions	Sacremental Association	Foods	Developmental Age Life Lesson
Sensitivity to pollution, chronic exhaustion, epilepsy, Alzheimer's	Depression, obsessional thinking, confusion	Extreme unction	(None) Fasting	(N/A) Selflessness
Headaches, poor vision, neurological disturbance, glaucoma	Nightmares, learning difficulties, hallucinations	Ordination	(None)	(N/A) Emotional intelligence
Sore throats, thyroid problems, hearing problems, tinnitus, asthma	Perfectionism, inability to express emotions, blocked creativity, incapable of stillness, difficulty achieving goals	Confession	Fruit	28-35 years Personal expression
Shallow breathing, high blood pressure, heart disease, cancer	Co-dependency, melancholia, fears concerning loneliness, commitment and/or betrayal	Marriage	Vegetable	21–28 years Forgiveness & compassion
Stomach ulcers, fatigue, weight around stomach, allergies, diabetes	Need to be in control, oversensitive to criticism, addictive personality, aggressiveness, low self-esteem	Confirmation	Complex carbohy-drates	14–21 years Self-esteem; self-confidence
Impotence, frigidity, bladder & prostate problems, lower back pain	Unbalanced sex drive, emotional instability, feelings of isolation	Communion	Liquids	8-14 yrs Challenging motivations based on social conditioning
Osteoarthritis	Mental lethargy, 'spaciness', incapable of inner stillness	Baptism	Proteins, meats	1–8 yrs Standing up for oneself

PART II

THE CHAKRAS

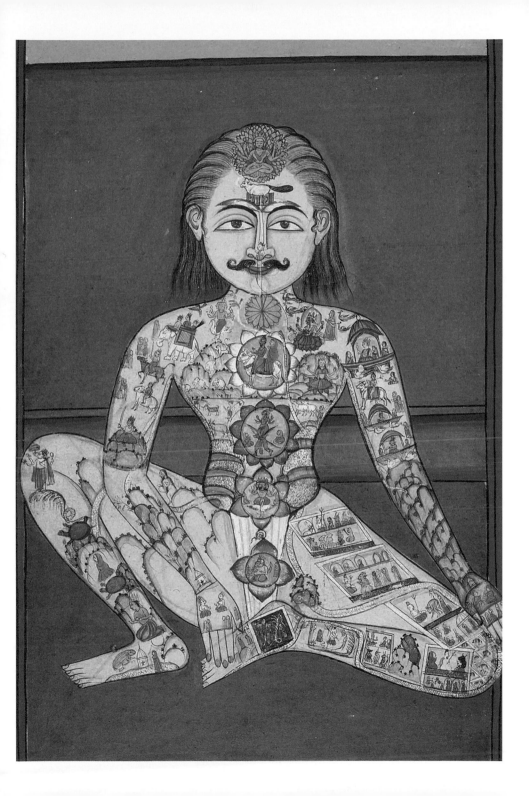

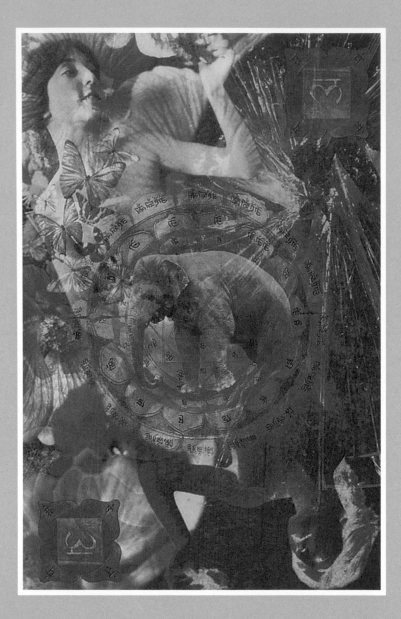

I THE ROOT CHAKRA: MULADHARA

The Root Chakra, or Muladhara, is also known as the root, adhara, mula, padma, brahma padma or bhumi chakra. It is the first of the seven major chakras and associated with the element of Earth, symbolizing the densest grade of manifestation and the basis of life.

In the kundalini yoga system of Shaktism, the Muladhara centre is described as having four lotus petals, blood-red in colour, each corresponding to the psychological states of greatest joy, natural pleasure, delight in controlling passions, and blissfulness in concentration, leading to meditation.

THE FUNCTIONS OF MULADHARA

In terms of energetics, this chakra channels Earth energy upwards through the feet and legs to process and stabilize it. It then moves the energy on, up the spine, now transmuted into a form that the body recognizes as signals, to balance the endocrine system (the gonads: ovaries and testes) through the release of hormones. When we do not get the full flow of this Earth energy, imbalances in our physical body result. 'Grounding' or 'rooting' us is the main function of

Muladhara. When we are grounded, we are at one with life and Muladhara functions as intended. We enter into a sympathetic vibration with the electromagnetic frequency of the Earth, coming into tune with the beat of 'her' heart.

Muladhara is also closely associated with returning karma – the sum of our experiences from previous existences. This is sometimes referred to as 'good' or 'bad' karma, but all karma is there for us to learn from, and we are fortunate if we believe that we get more than one chance at life!

The first and second chakras also act as the energetic recycling bin of the auric field. They change negative emotional energies into power and light, and return to Earth any 'toxic waste' that the other chakras are unable to deal with, thus keeping the rainbow purity of the aura. If our Muladhara chakra is disassociated from the Earth, we cannot expel these waste emotions.

ROOT CHAKRA CORRESPONDENCES

This chart for the Root (First) Chakra identifies all the associations and symbolisms linked with this particular chakra. As such it provides a 'ready reference' of inspirations to use when you carry out practical exercises such as choosing appropriate stones for crystal work.

USING THE CHART

This chart will also help you with the various images that you will need when composing your own meditations and visualizations. Incorporate as many of these symbols and themes as you feel is appropriate to your needs.

By reacquainting yourself regularly with this chakra chart as a prelude to the section on the Root Chakra, you will help to keep your mind focused on related issues, including an awareness of your physical body and your survival needs through diet, exercise, and interactions with the 'tribe', or group identity.

Mastering the Root Chakra helps you grasp the importance of a fit, healthy body as you travel upward through higher and higher levels of consciousness.

CHAKRA CHARACTERISTICS

See which of the following characteristics of excessive ('too open'), deficient ('blocked'), and balanced chakra energy you can relate to – and then determine (should you choose) to take the necessary action, using the tools and techniques outlined in this following pages of this chapter.

- **Too open** (chakra spins too fast): bullying, overly materialistic, self-centred, engages in physical foolhardiness.

- **Blocked** (chakra spins sluggishly or not at all): emotionally needy, low self-esteem, self-destructive behaviour, fearful.

- **Balanced** (chakra maintains equilibrium and spins at correct vibrational speed): demonstrates self-mastery, high physical energy, grounded, healthy.

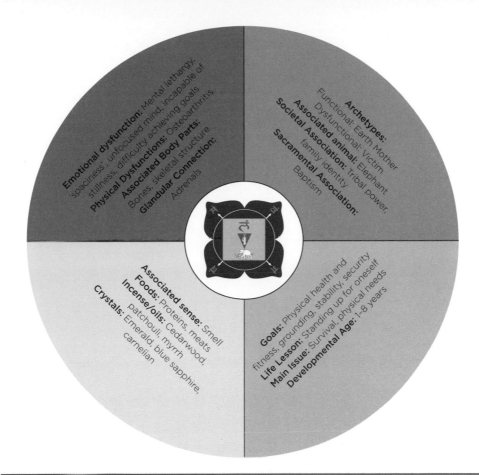

Archetypes:
Functional: Earth Mother
Dysfunctional: Victim
Associated animal: Elephant
Societal Association: Tribal power,
family identity
Sacramental Association:
Baptism

Goals: Physical health and
fitness, grounding, stability, security
Life Lesson: Standing up for oneself
Main Issue: Survival, physical needs
Developmental Age: 1–8 years

Associated sense: Smell
Foods: Proteins, meats
Incense/oils: Cedarwood,
patchouli, myrrh
Crystals: Emerald, blue sapphire,
carnelian

Emotional dysfunction: Mental lethargy,
'spaciness', unfocused mind, incapable of
stillness, difficulty achieving goals
Physical Dysfunctions: Osteoarthritis
Associated Body Parts:
Bones, skeletal structure
Glandular Connection:
Adrenals

ROOT CHAKRA	
Sanskrit name	Muladhara
Meaning	Root or support
Location	Base of spine, between anus and genitals
Symbol	Four red petals around a square containing a downward-pointing triangle (see page 50 for the yantra).
Associated colour	Red
Element	Earth
Ruling planet	Saturn

ROOT CHAKRA YANTRA

*In this lotus is the square of Earth, surrounded by eight
shining spears. It is shining yellow and beautiful like lightning,
as the seed-sound Lam, which is within.*

— Sat Cakra Nirupana, a Sanskrit text written c. 1577

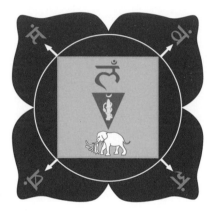

YANTRA DESCRIPTION

- **Number of petals:** The Muladhara
yantra has four petals, symbolizing
the four directions and four
qualities of bliss.

- **Colour:** The colour most associated
with the Muladhara yantra is red.
Four red petals surround a yellow
square. The square represents
Earth, the element that is
associated with this chakra.

- **White elephant:** Airavata, the
white elephant, reminds us of
our instinctive animal nature.
The elephant is a strong and
intelligent animal, but has
destructive tendencies, too. This is
a dilemma that often confronts us
in Muladhara. The white elephant
has seven trunks, each of which
symbolizes one of the seven
elements that are considered
essential for physical life.

- **Trikona:** The triangular shape
at the centre of the Muladhara
yantra represents Shakti, (female)
energy. The lingam, or phallus,
within the triangle represents male,
Shiva energy. Kundalini energy is
depicted as a serpent wrapped
around the lingam.

- **Crescent moon:** The crescent moon
that crowns the lingam within the
triangle, symbolizes the Divine
source of all energy.

ROOT CHAKRA ARCHETYPES

The Root (First) Chakra is associated with physical security. Our earliest experiences, including the extent to which our basic needs were met, or not, when infants, are recorded and stored there – like a message on a magnetic tape. Our emotional security comes from a sense of belonging to a group, and this aspect of our psychological well-being relates to the Root Chakra.

The archetypes associated with the Root Chakra are the Victim and the Earth Mother. They represent two sides of the same coin – the positive face and our darker side.

THE VICTIM

Dysfunctional Victims are increasingly commonplace as people look for others to blame for their problems. If you are a Victim you allow yourself to become vulnerable, needy, and hence ungrounded, because you regard every disappointment, separation, or loss as something that you cannot control or change. Subconsciously you may still consider yourself to be the baby who can't get up and feed itself and so has to rely on others. Only by recognizing that you have the power to provide everything you need for yourself can you reframe your experiences into opportunities for self-sufficiency, strength, and emotional wholeness. Changing this

negative archetype involves taking responsibility for your life, accepting that you have choices and deserve the best that life has to offer.

THE EARTH MOTHER

The functional side of this archetype is the Earth Mother, universally associated with nourishment, caring, and unconditional love. By recognizing the Earth Mother within you (regardless of gender) you acknowledge that you are capable of providing all the physical and emotional security you need for yourself, by yourself. You can begin to develop this ability in a practical way by attending to your inner child's needs, by keeping your home environment safe and comforting, by treating yourself in a motherly way from time to time, and affirming that there is nothing you cannot accomplish, either single-handedly or by asking others for help.

ROOT CHAKRA AROMATHERAPY

Our sense of smell is acute and can distinguish between those smells that we call bad or offensive and those that give us pleasure. Perfumed oils have been used since the earliest times: by 3500 BCE priestesses in Egyptian temples were burning tree gums and resins such as frankincense to clear the air and mind; ancient Greeks and the Egyptians were skilled at blending all manner of herbs in fatty-paste pomanders for the treatment of wounds and cosmetics; and the Romans used fragrant oils for massage.

It was brilliant Arab physicians who were among the first to build up the most comprehensive knowledge of the therapeutic properties of plants. By the 12th century the 'perfumes of Arabia' were being brought back to Europe by knight crusaders, although the knowledge of how to distil them remained unknown in Europe for many more centuries.

In the first decade of the 20th century a French chemist, René Maurice Gattefosse, and Dr Jean Valnet began to make essential oils. During the First World War, Valnet used them to successfully treat severe burns, battle injuries and psychiatric problems.

ESSENTIAL OILS

Essential oils that have a sympathetic resonance with Muladhara are:

- **Cedarwood:** This comes from steam distillation of the wood. It is antiseptic, anti-seborrhoeic, astringent, diuretic, emmenagogic, expectorant, sedative and an insecticide.

- **Patchouli:** This oil is steam-distilled from dried, fermented leaves and is very popular in India and the Far East. It acts as an anti-depressant, anti-inflammatory, anti-microbial, antiseptic, aphrodisiac, deodorant, sedative and an insecticide.

- **Myrrh:** This is derived from a shrubby tree that produces a brown resin from the bark. It is sedative, antiseptic, astringent, carminative, expectorant and anti-inflammatory.

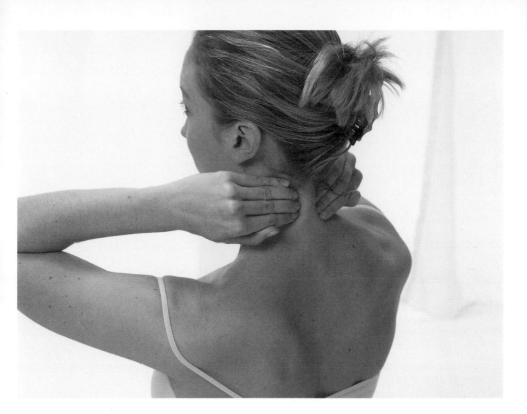

SIMPLE AROMATHERAPY MASSAGE

This massage is easy to perform on yourself.

1 Refer to pages 28–30 for instructions on mixing essential oils with a base oil. Sit on the floor comfortably, covered with a towel. Remove all clothing from your upper body and expose your neck.

2 Warm a little oil in your hands and massage over your neck and shoulder areas, gradually increasing the pressure.

3 Work the muscles of each shoulder firmly, making small friction circles wherever you feel deep-seated tension.

4 Position your fingertips behind your head on either side of your neck, then make friction circles as you work gradually up, and then down the neck muscles.

Caution: Essential oils should never be used on babies and children under 12 years of age. During pregnancy their use is limited to a few safe oils. It is best to seek advice from an aromatherapist.

YOGA FOR THE ROOT CHAKRA

Start your yoga session by balancing the chakras with a standing balanced asana (posture) such as Pranamasana (prayer pose). This is simply standing straight with the spine 'lifted', as if a cord is pulling it up from the crown of your head, and placing your hands together in the prayer position.

ACTIVE ASANA: WARRIOR

This strong standing asana makes a firm connection with the prana coming into your Root Chakra. Physically it strengthens your legs and benefits your back. The state of consciousness associated with Muladhara is annamayakosha (deep sleep), which is experienced through the physical body. As you use your breath to move you in a light, fluid way into this asana, visualize it being red in colour.

1 Stand with your feet about 1 m (3 ft) apart. Turn your right foot to the right, and bend your right knee until it is in line with your ankle.

2 Keeping your back straight, stretch both arms above your head, bringing the palms of your hands together. Repeat on the opposite side.

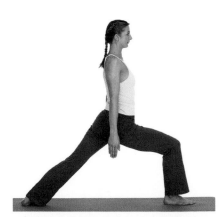

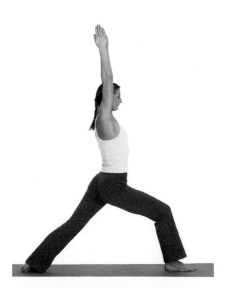

ACTIVE ASANA: TRIANGLE

The strong triangle shape of the legs in this pose is symbolic of the movement of Earth energy upwards through the chakras, which begins with the Root Chakra.

It complements the downward-pointed triangle of cosmic energy depicted in the Muladhara yantra. Thus you start a journey to understand the symbolism of the interlocking triangle that you will encounter at the Heart Chakra.

The physical and subtle-energy benefits of this pose are similar to those of The Warrior.

As with the Warrior, visualize your breath being red in colour as you use it to move you in a light, fluid way into this asana.

1 Stand with your legs wider than your shoulders, making an equilateral triangle with the floor. Raise both arms to your sides, level with your shoulders.

2 Turn your left foot out, slowly bend to the left and take a firm hold of your left ankle with your left hand. Your neck should be relaxed, with your head falling sideways. Your right arm should be stretched over your head, parallel with the floor. Repeat on the opposite side.

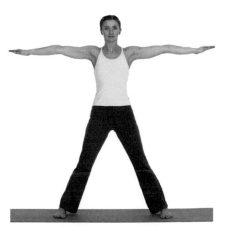

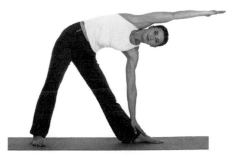

PASSIVE ASANA: EAGLE

The Eagle is the penultimate asana in the sequence of asanas to benefit the energies of the chakras, and demonstrates that you have come to a state of inner stillness and balance. It benefits the knees, ankles and shoulders, and helps to prevent cramp in the calf muscles. A gentle and peaceful type of energy is now locked within the sexual organs as you maintain this balance to complete your yoga practice.

1 Stand upright with your feet together and your hands at your sides. Bend your right knee, bringing it over the left knee and tucking the right foot behind the left calf. Balance in this position.

2 Now bend your elbows in front of you and entwine your arms, so that the right elbow rests on the front of the left arm's inner elbow. Join the palms of your hands together. Maintain your balance. Repeat with the opposite leg and arm.

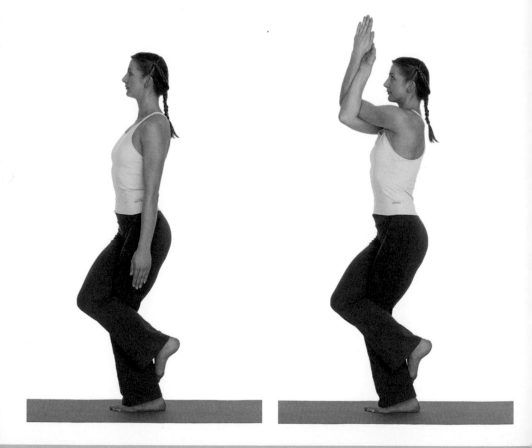

CRYSTALS TO CALM THE ROOT CHAKRA

Recommended gemstone crystals for calming the Root Chakra are small, uncut pieces of emerald or blue sapphire. To achieve clarity about spiritual matters, use blue sapphire to enable a connection to be made with your spiritual origins, ancestral roots and cosmic origins.

EMERALD

Emerald, when used on the Root Chakra, will calm it by bringing you into a deeper resonance with Mother Earth. Emerald helps to ground us, so that we feel much more at peace with our lives on Earth. It is vital that we are all grounded through our Root Chakra, since unless we are, the other chakras will not be fully in alignment with our soul purpose.

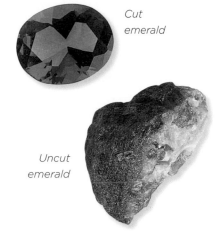

Cut emerald

Uncut emerald

Using emerald to ground yourself
Arrange not to be disturbed for at least 30 minutes.

1 In a cross-legged meditation pose, sit on the floor on your emerald! (If you don't want to actually sit on it, hold it in your non-dominant hand at your Root Chakra). If you sense that you need a lot of grounding, put a dense stone under each foot as well.

2 Now relax, but keep your spine straight, visualizing roots growing out from under your feet:

first a strong 'tap root', then smaller roots in a network of finer and finer filaments, working their way through the earth, rocks and stones. Your roots are so powerful that they can pass around any obstacles in their way and eventually connect to the crystalline heart of Mother Earth at the centre of the planet.

3 Come slowly back to everyday awareness.

CRYSTALS TO BALANCE THE ROOT CHAKRA

A popular New Age myth is that a set of seven 'chakra stones' of different colours will balance your chakras. They might be effective, but healers who specialize in using crystals use different crystals for specific purposes.

This book recommends several precious gemstones to activate or calm each chakra.

In addition we suggest a number of less precious stones to balance out the energies and bring harmony – these stones can be 'tumble-polished' so that they end up looking like smooth pebbles.

CRYSTAL HEALING

A crystal healer will generally only work on one or two of the chakras at a time: you should never overload someone's body or auric field with the power of crystals.

Instead, it is far better to ascertain the lowest chakra that is out of balance and work upon it. Check that it is balanced to optimum levels before proceeding to the next chakra up. When all the chakras are balanced, they come into a state called 'harmonization'.

To check the state of your chakras, try the following techniques:

• See of you can sense them using your hands.

• Try to visualize the condition of the chakra in your mind's eye.

• Using a pendulum.

• Try to asses the condition of your chakras clairvoyantly (if you happen to be gifted in this way).

CARNELIAN

A small carnelian pebble/tumbled stone (or black tourmaline) is ideal for balancing Muladhara. And, provided you have consulted a doctor about any acutely painful condition, you can use a flat, polished carnelian, taped into position over the problem area, for pain reduction. Remove the carnelian at least three times a day and cleanse it by washing.

Using carnelian to balance yourself

Create a quiet and clear 'sacred space' around yourself, then begin.

1 Sit quietly in a chair with a straight back and your bare feet flat on the floor. Have your carnelian ready cleansed (see page 36) and close by.

2 Let your breath flow deeply into your body, and ground yourself (see page 38).

3 Close your eyes and visualize the condition of each chakra in turn, working upwards. Notice what colours and energies you see. Are the energies still or moving?

4 Now return to the Root Chakra: this is the one you are going to balance with the carnelian.

5 Holding the carnelian in your non-dominant hand, visualize the Root Chakra again. Ask for it to come into balance. You can even talk to it – and thank it when it seems balanced.

6 Allow yourself to come back slowly and gently to everyday awareness. Take your time.

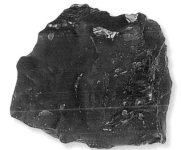

Uncut carnelian

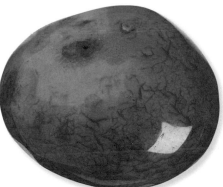

Cut carnelian

CRYSTAL VISUALIZATION

Yantras are symbols that are used to represent each chakra and can be a useful meditation tool (see pages 24–25). They are the yogi equivalent of the Buddhist mandala: visual symbols of complex spiritual concepts. Each chakra yantra is based on a lotus, the traditional symbol of enlightenment in Hindu and Buddhist thought.

For this crystal visualization you ideally need three small pieces of black tourmaline, although one will do. You are going to root yourself into the collective unconscious mind of humanity.

1 Turn off your phone and make sure you will not be disturbed. Allow about 30 minutes for this exercise.

2 Sit in an upright chair, in a cross-legged yoga posture or lie down. Take your shoes and socks off.

3 Your tourmaline should already be cleansed (see page 36). Place one piece underneath your spine and sit on it (if you have only one tourmaline, put it here); rest the other pieces in the palm of each hand.

4 Begin to breathe deeply. Do this for some minutes.

5 Be aware of the ground beneath you, and start to visualize a strong root growing from the bottom of your spine out through the soles of your feet.

6 Imagine that you are a tiny seed full of life-force energy. Tiny rootlets are growing from your spinal root, seeking nourishment in the Earth. They are looking for water. Your task is to see the network of roots taking up water, passing it into your body through the Root Chakra.

7 Now see your spine as the trunk of a tree. Check that your body is perfectly balanced on either side of your spine.

8 Visualize your head in the element of air. Now you can see yourself fully as a tree with roots, trunk and branches.

9 Look closely at the branches: What type of leaves do they have? Do they have flowers or fruit on them? Accept whatever you see.

10 Now focus inwardly, realizing that you draw nourishment from the Earth, just like a tree. In the world of energy vibration, nothing is separate: you and the tree are one.

11 When ready to finish, breathe more deeply. Let go of the tree visualization. Reach down to your feet and rub them, then rub your legs.

12 Hold all your crystals in the palms of your hands and, breathing on them, thank them for their energy.

13 Stretch your body, remembering that you are a tree reaching up to the light.

Keep notes of your experience.

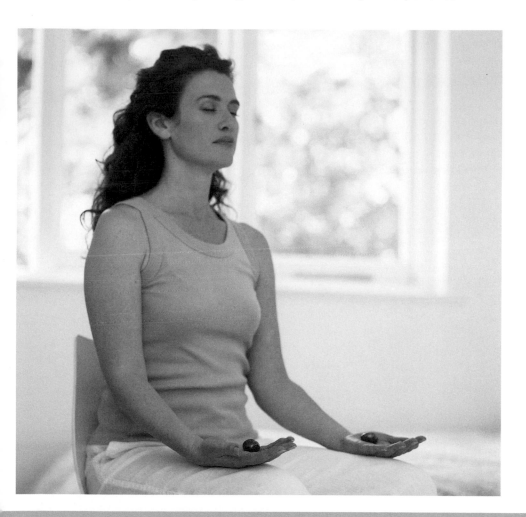

ROOT CHAKRA MEDITATION

A good time for meditation is either following yoga practise or after crystal therapy. At such times, your body is already relaxed and ready for a session of focused concentration (see pages 22–23).

BEFORE YOU START

Choose a leisurely and relaxed time to meditate. If you like, create an atmosphere with oils, candles, or incense in the colour of the chakra. Sit or lie somewhere you won't be disturbed. You can pre-record the words of the meditation – dots indicate a pause.

1 Breathe slowly and deeply through your nose.

2 Tense each set of muscles in turn, from feet to head ... then relax them, gradually sinking into the floor or chair ...

3 Visualize yourself in perfect surroundings. You are safe, warm, and secure.

4 Who are the people in this happy place with you? Acknowledge each one ... Feel their love radiate as a reddish golden glow penetrating every cell of your being, filling you with joy ...

AFFIRMATIONS

• My body is becoming more important to me. I nurture my body constantly.

• I am taking responsibility for my life. I can cope with any situation that comes my way.

• I recognize the abundance of love, trust, and care surrounding me.

• My internal mother is always here for me, protecting, nourishing, and soothing me.

• I deserve the very best that life has to offer. My needs are always met.

• I am connected to Mother Earth and know the security of being grounded in reality, in the moment.

5 Imagine your inner mother looking benevolently down on you. Sense her smile enveloping you like a soft cloak ... Know that she will never let you down. She is part of you and will always protect you.

6 Approach your inner mother. Hug, kiss, or link arms. Enjoy the sensation ... Take time to get to know one another. Enjoy the sensation of re-acquaintance and trust ...

7 She gives you a present. Examine it closely ... Thank your mother and tell her you will treasure her gift. It is yours to keep and recall every time you feel victimized.

8 As you hold your gift, feel the energy of your inner mother's love channelled into your Root Chakra ... Imagine this chakra as a four-petalled lotus rotating rhythmically like a wheel ...

9 Focus on the smooth motion of the chakra and the warm, red glow that fills that part of your body, flowing down your legs to connect you with the Earth ...

10 Enjoy the reassuring sensation of groundedness, security, and stability before bringing your attention back to your everyday surroundings.

DAILY QUESTIONS

- Does your home reflect who you are? If not, how can you change it?

- What reward have you given yourself today? A gift, an affirmation, praise, or good turn?

- Have you focused on abundance or lack today? List things representing abundance (family support/money saved).

- How could you improve financial security? List weekly expenses. Where could savings be made?

- Have you lost contact with family or friends? How could you re-establish links? (Make approaches through love, not obligation.)

- How do you honour your body? Do you address diet, exercise, and relaxation regularly?

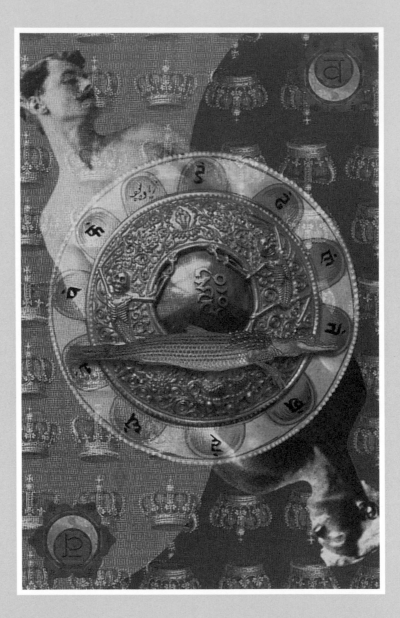

2 THE SACRAL CHAKRA: SVADHISTHANA

The Sacral Chakra, or Svadisthana, is also known as the spleen and navel centre, adhishthana, bhima, shatpatra, skaddala padma, wari-chakra and medhra. In the Indian Tantric tradition, Svadisthana can be translated as 'one's sweetest abode' or 'one's own place'.

In the kundalini yoga system of Shaktism, Svadisthana is described as having six lotus petals, which symbolize its secret connection with the high Sixth State of Consciousness into which we are evolving. The petals are associated with: all-destructiveness, affection, pitilessness, a feeling of delusion, disdain, and suspicion on the path to the Sixth State.

This second chakra corresponds to the element of Water and is traditionally associated with sexual energy. It does not correspond with the sex organs (these are the function of Muhadhara), but to the original life-sustaining energy behind sexual impulse.

THE FUNCTIONS OF SVADISTHANA

Indian teachings place a great deal of emphasis on celibacy, in order to raise and transmute powerful sexual energy, passing it to the brain (or, more correctly, the Upper Tan Tien Centre, to use the Taoist paradigm) and thereby increasing higher consciousness. This is actually the basic principle behind celibacy in all religions (including Catholicism). In practice, though, this noble ideal often flounders, because someone who is not ready to renounce physical sex may become psychologically unbalanced and full of guilt, or turn to paedophilia or other unnatural forms of sex.

ASSIMILATION

When Svadisthana is fully developed, it produces the necessary radiance to unite in a bond of love with another soul and fuels the growth of consciousness to enlightenment. Because this chakra is concerned with assimilation – of sexual expression and food, as well as ideas and creativity – it is often referred to as the centre of self-expression.

SACRAL CHAKRA CORRESPONDENCES

This chart for the Sacral (Second) Chakra provides a 'ready reference' of inspirations to use when you carry out practical exercises such choosing appropriate stones for crystal work. It will also help you with the various images you will need when composing your own meditations and visualizations. Incorporate as many of these symbols and themes as are appropriate to your needs.

USING THE CHART

By re-acquainting yourself regularly with this chakra chart as a prelude to the section on the Sacral Chakra, you will help to keep your mind focused on related issues. This includes an acceptance of the desire to enjoy a pleasurable lifestyle and to embrace whatever change is necessary to bring that about.

Finding pleasure in life's activities generates the enthusiasm and energy to take on even more creative projects, whether concerning family, business, relationships, or social activities. This is what the Sacral Chakra can bring you.

CHAKRA CHARACTERISTICS

See which of the following characteristics of excessive ('too open'), deficient ('blocked'), and balanced chakra energy you can related to - and then determine (should you choose) to take the necessary action, using the tools and techniques outlined in this chapter.

- **Too open** (chakra spins too fast): emotionally unbalanced, a fantasist, manipulative, sexually addictive.

- **Blocked** (chakra spins sluggishly or not at all): over-sensitive, hard on him/herself, feels guilty for no reason, frigid or impotent.

- **Balanced** (chakra maintains equilibrium and spins at correct vibrational speed): trusting, expressive, attuned to his/her own feelings, creative.

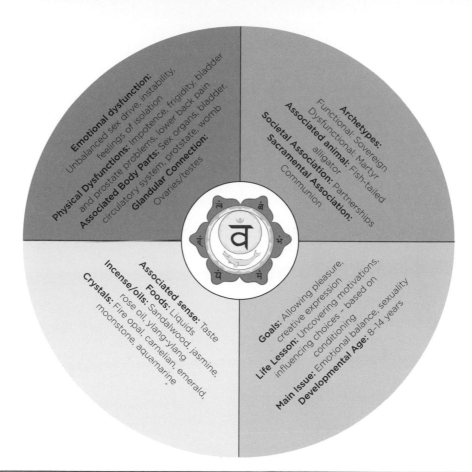

Emotional dysfunction: Unbalanced sex drive, instability, feelings of isolation.
Physical Dysfunctions: Impotence, frigidity, bladder and prostate problems, lower back pain
Associated Body Parts: Sex organs, bladder, circulatory system, protstate, womb
Glandular Connection: Ovaries/testes

Archetypes:
Functional: Sovereign
Dysfunctional: Martyr
Associated animal: Fish-tailed alligator
Societal Association: Partnerships
Sacramental Association: Communion

Associated sense: Taste
Foods: Liquids
Incense/oils: Sandalwood, jasmine, rose oil, ylang-ylang
Crystals: Fire opal, carnelian, emerald, moonstone, aquamarine .

Goals: Allowing pleasure, creative expression
Life Lesson: Uncovering motivations, influencing choices – based on conditioning
Main Issue: Emotional balance, sexuality
Developmental Age: 8-14 years

SACRAL CHAKRA	
Sanskrit name	Svadhisthana
Meaning	Sweetness
Location	Lower abdomen, between navel and genitals
Symbol	Six orange-red petals containing a second lotus flower and a crescent moon (see page 68 for the yantra).
Associated colour	Orange
Element	Water
Ruling planet	Pluto

SACRAL CHAKRA YANTRA

Within Svadisthana is the white, shining, watery region of the shape of a half moon, stainless and white as the autumnal moon. He who meditates upon this stainless Lotus is free immediately from all his enemies (Kama – lust, Krodha – anger, Lobha – greed, Moha – delusion, Matsaryya – envy).

— Sat Cakra Nirupana

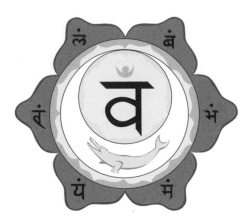

DESCRIPTION OF THE YANTRA

- **Number of petals:** The Svadisthana yantra has six petals, shown variously as white, saffron or orange in colour.

- **Colour:** The colour of the Svadisthana yantra is usually vermilion in the ancient texts, but more generally depicted as orange today.

- **Element:** The element associated with Svadisthana is Water, the essence of life.

- **Crescent moon:** The Svadisthana yantra has a crescent moon in the centre. This is the tattwa (truth) of water and it symbolizes regeneration. The crescent moon is also symbolic of the mysterious powers hiding within the unconscious mind and relates to the pre-rational dream state of consciousness.

- **Makara:** Towards the bottom of the Svadisthana yantra lies the mythical fish-tailed alligator, known as Makara. The serpentine movement of this creature reflects the sensuous aspects of someone dominated by their second chakra. The fish-tailed alligator, or Makara, is also associated with sexual power. Legend has it that the fat of the creature was once used as an aid to male virility.

SACRAL CHAKRA ARCHETYPES

The Sacral (Second) Chakra further develops the themes of the Root (First) Chakra of personal responsibility and self-expression. Its archetypes are the Sovereign and the Martyr, which are concerned with our attitudes concerning abundance and how much we believe that we deserve to enjoy life.

These two associations represent the polarities of pleasure and fulfilment, and suffering and sacrifice.

THE MARTYR

Martyrs are less likely than Victims to blame external influences for what they perceive as a life of suffering, but share a similar belief that they don't deserve better. Martyrdom involves being entrenched in a pit of self-pity with no motivation to shift the negative attitudes contributing to the situation. Martyrs' lives are steeped in a sense of lack, which underpins a justification for not changing behaviours because there is just not enough good fortune in the world to go round - and they have drawn the short straw. So they complain, but never take any action. Theirs is a passive acceptance of life rather than the active desire to change. Without a proper regard for personal needs and desires, mothers very often develop into Martyrs.

THE SOVEREIGN

The Sovereign allows the good things of life to be part of their everyday experiences. These individuals do not necessarily live charmed lives, it's simply that when confronted with a challenging situation they see the positive opportunities for growth and development. They are content to take the rough with the smooth in the knowledge that life is all about shades of light and dark, positives and negatives, good and bad. Nurturing their own desires is a high priority for Sovereigns. To them, they, as much as anyone else, deserve a share in the rewards that surround them, including sexual fulfilment. Sex to them is something to be celebrated and enjoyed. Taking a creative approach to their sexuality, Sovereigns achieve fulfilment in this important area of their lives. Because they are always looking out for the benefits rather than disadvantages, they tend to find that that's exactly what life offers to them.

SACRAL CHAKRA AROMATHERAPY

There are numerous herbs, plants and flower essences that will benefit the Svadisthana Chakra. Red clover, currant, fennel, grapefruit and onion are among the most effective.

SACRAL CHAKRA ESSENTIAL OILS

The main essential oils that have a sympathetic resonance with Svadisthana are:

- **Sandalwood:** This oil has a vibrational correspondence with Svadisthana. It comes from an evergreen tropical tree, and the essential oil is steam-distilled from the heartwood and roots. The oil is anti-depressant, anti-septic, anti-spasmodic, aphrodisiac, astringent, bactericide, sedative and expectorant.

- **Jasmine:** This is a beautiful flowering shrub, whose strong perfume is produced by solvent extraction. It is analgesic, anti-depressant, anti-inflammatory, antiseptic, aphrodisiac, sedative and uterine.

- **Rose oil:** This is obtained by solvent extraction or steam distillation. It takes around 30 perfect and specially cultivated rose blooms to make just one drop of essential oil. Its main use with the Sacral Chakra is as an aphrodisiac, although it is also regarded as anti-depressant, antiseptic, emmenagogic, hepatic, sedative and uterine.

- **Ylang-ylang:** These flowers come from a tropical tree called the cananga. It is a voluptuous, exotic perfume and is used as an aphrodisiac. It is also anti-depressant, antiseptic and sedative. Its use will help dispel anger held at the Sacral Chakra area.

- **Champaca:** This is a lesser-known exotic oil from India, which is obtained by solvent extraction. It is aphrodisiac, anti-depressant and stimulant.

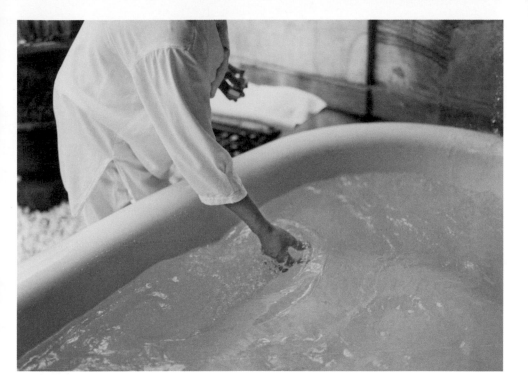

AROMATIC BATHING

It can be very enjoyable to explore sensuality with exotic oils. Warm bath water helps you to relax and absorb the oils, so it is excellent to bathe before going to bed. Any of the oils mentioned opposite are suitable.

1 Run a bath of warm (not too hot) water and, when it is ready, add a maximum of five drops of essential oil (5 ml) – these drops can be a combination of several oils.

2 Mix the water with your hands, then relax in it for a while.

3 Make your bath more of a special occasion by lighting several candles associated with the colour of the chakra (in this case, orange). You can float the appropriate flowers in the water too.

Cautions: Avoid getting any of the bath water in your eyes – rinse immediately if this happens. Vary the essential oils you use with each bath, so that you do not risk a build-up of any one type in your body. Consult an aromatherapist if you are pregnant. Do not use essential oils for children under 12 years of age, even in the bath, unless with qualified supervision.

YOGA FOR THE SACRAL CHAKRA

Start your yoga session by balancing the chakras with a standing balanced asana (posture) such as Pranamasana (prayer pose). This is simply standing straight with the spine 'lifted', as if a cord is pulling it up from the crown of your head, and placing your hands together in the prayer position.

ACTIVE ASANA: TWISTING TRIANGLE

The Twisting Triangle has the same effect on energy flows as the Root Chakra asanas, but the twisting movement helps to focus energy in the region of the Sacral Chakra. As you 'breathe into' this asana, visualize orange-coloured light coming into your lungs to help you.

1 Stand with your feet about 1 m (3 ft) apart. Turn your right foot 90 degrees to the right, so that your body faces right, with your left foot only slightly turned to act as a base. Rotate your body towards your right leg, reaching down to the ankle or to the floor with your left hand beyond your right foot (advanced position).

2 Stretch your right arm straight up until it is in a direct line with the left arm. Repeat on the opposite side.

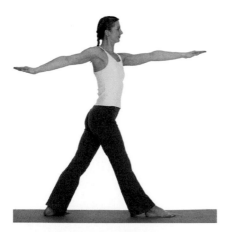
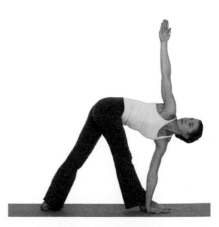

ACTIVE ASANA: EXTENDED LATERAL ANGLE POSE

This asana stretches every part of the body, but especially the hamstrings and spine. The chest, hips and legs should be in a line in order to do this. The Svadisthana region becomes the centre of balance, and so energy is focused there and can then flow uninterrupted through the spine and the associated nadis. The state of consciousness associated with the Sacral Chakra is pranamaya kosha (dream sleep). As with other chakras, you can use the yantra or appropriate coloured light as your focus.

1 Stand with your feet together and your arms stretched above your head. Now jump your feet about 1.5 m (5 ft) apart. Raise your arms sideways to shoulder level. Turn your left foot sideways 90 degrees to the left, keeping your right leg stretched and tight at the knee. Bend your left knee to make 90-degree angle.

2 Place your left palm flat on the floor by your left foot and stretch your right arm over your right ear. Look upwards, to the ceiling. Feel both your spine and the side of your body stretch as you move. Repeat on the opposite side.

PASSIVE ASANA: POSE OF SHIVA

The Pose of Shiva represents the dancing form of Lord Shiva, a symbolic synthesis of the most important aspects of Hinduism and the Vedas. The pose is performed most beautifully by ballerinas and ice-dancers. It makes your legs strong and supple. It requires the utmost concentration to perform it for some minutes, and during this concentration the focus should be on the Sacral Chakra region. It is this area that will begin to 'ground' you again (energetically speaking) after your yoga practice. You may use the yantra illustration, placed a little distance away on the floor in front of you. If you are practising outdoors, your gaze in this asana would normally be towards the horizon.

1 Stand and balance on your left foot, while simultaneously raising your left arm above your head. Bend your right knee and lift it behind you, until your right hand can hold the right foot. Relax and maintain your balance for a few moments.

2 Lift your right foot higher and stretch your left arm forwards. Relax and maintain your balance. Repeat with the opposite leg.

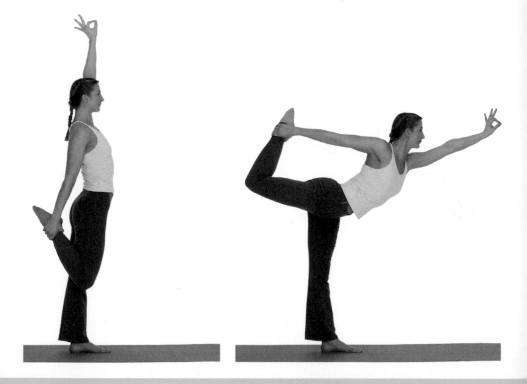

CRYSTALS TO ACTIVATE THE SACRAL CHAKRA

The main gemstone crystals used to activate the Sacral Chakra are fire opal and carnelian. Other crystals that you could use are humble orange calcite and scintillating yellow topaz.

Orange calcite works at a basic physical level. Its action is cleansing. It also balances the emotions, inspiring confidence. Yellow topaz will cause the movement of energetic imbalances on elevated spiritual levels through this chakra, after using orange calcite for the physical levels.

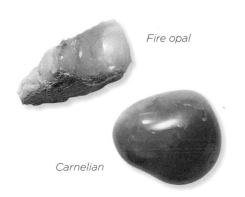

Fire opal

Carnelian

FIRE OPAL

Fire opal has a large water content, but sparkles with flashes of red 'fire'. It stimulates creativity. Psychologically, it is said to move emotional blockages because of its association with water. Conversely, in many ways its fiery nature is quite apparent and intensifies the manifestation of our own inner fire: negatively as anger, or positively by moving the Sacral Chakra into enjoyment of our own sexuality, leading to enlightenment as radiance moves through the kundalini channel. Healers may choose fire opal for energetic imbalances of the kidneys and blood, aiding purification. It is beneficial for the eyes when used as a crystal essence/elixir. Opal has been gifted to us by the Earth in many different colours, each of which has specific healing properties.

CARNELIAN

This gemstone varies in colour from pink through to deep orange. It has a strong influence on the Sacral Chakra. For this reason it is recommended to energetically balance lower back problems, rheumatism and arthritis. It also assists the kidneys to regulate their water energies.

CRYSTALS TO CALM THE SACRAL CHAKRA

Emerald is regarded as 'the stone of fulfilled love'; it encourages friendship, calms the emotions and brings wisdom. Emeralds were once worn to protect from epilepsy – a frightening condition when not understood. They were also believed to be an antidote to poison, an 'occupational hazard' in medieval times, when kings would wear an emerald ring for this reason.

EMERALD AND SVADISTHANA

The colour and vibration of emerald are generally calming to Svadisthana. You can obtain small pieces of uncut emerald, which are inexpensive, or a much pricier cut gem.

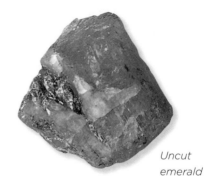

Uncut emerald

Whether a crystal is large or small makes no difference to the type of energy it holds; it still has the same vibration whether it is one carat or ten. However, there will be more available energy if it is larger. Cut and polished gems transmit more light through them than uncut ones or less precious stones.

If you cannot obtain emerald, then green-coloured denser stones will be appropriate to calm an overenergized Svadisthana. Try using green aventurine, amazonite or green calcite, if the energy imbalance is connected with a physical body condition manifesting as 'dis-ease' or mental anguish.

You will need to send a lot of unconditional love to begin to shift the problem. As a general rule, first begin to heal the physical body, then work at subtle levels of the aura and chakra system. For this reason, crystals that operate at a vibrational level should not be used as a replacement for medical attention.

You do not have to be undressed for crystals to be effective, but it helps to be wearing white natural cotton when you undergo a crystal healing.

Using emerald to calm yourself

This meditation involves making a small layout of crystals as follows over the sacral region.

1 Cleanse and dedicate all the crystals you will use (see pages 36–38).

2 Carefully place an emerald at the centre of the Sacral Chakra.

3 Arrange six small, clear quartz pointed crystals, pointing inwards, in a circle around the emerald (see photograph below).

4 Wait in relaxed meditation mode for at least ten minutes for the chakra to become calmer. After this time, you may sense that it is time to remove the crystals.

5 Allow yourself to come back slowly and gently to everyday awareness. Take your time.

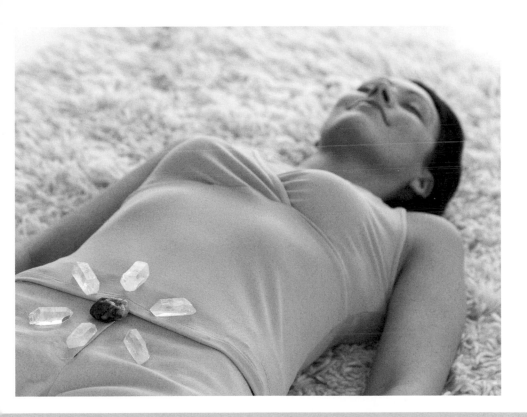

CRYSTALS TO BALANCE
THE SACRAL CHAKRA

Moonstone and aquamarine are ideal for using at the Sacral Chakra because of their associations with the element of Water. Moonstone has traditionally been valued to ease insomnia and develop psychic abilities. It works particularly with the feminine energy impulse.

AQUAMARINE

Aquamarine is regarded as giving strength in adversity and was traditionally believed to protect against the forces of evil. From a spiritual healing perspective, it aligns our physical body with the whole of our subtle-energy field. Energetically, it works to cleanse the kidneys and genitourinary system.

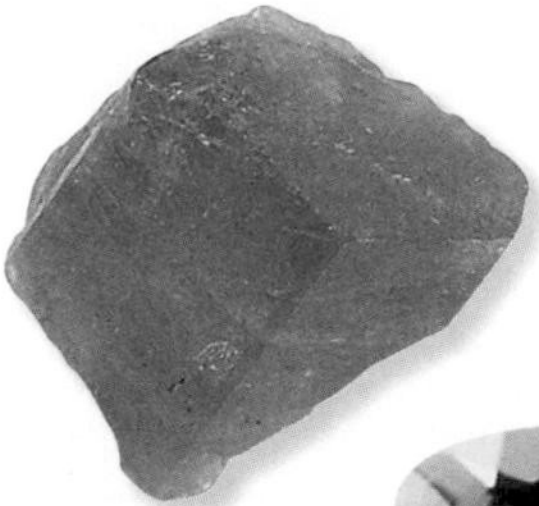

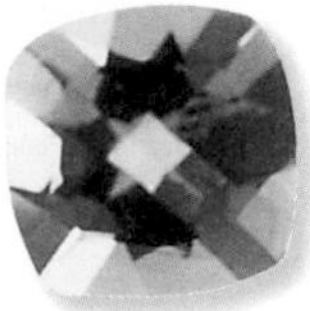

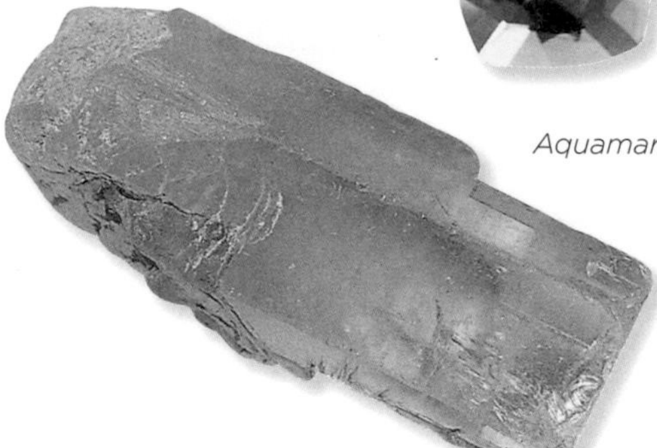

Aquamarine

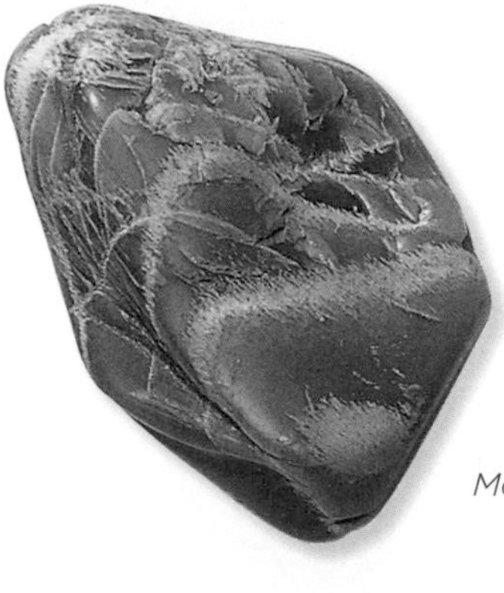

Moonstone

MAKING A CRYSTAL ESSENCE BY THE DIRECT METHOD

A crystal essence (or gem elixir) affects the mind, body and spirit – as do flower essences and homeopathic remedies. However, crystal essences generally affect the physical body more effectively than flower essences, but less effectively than homeopathic remedies.

Any crystal that is hard enough to be tumble-polished can be used to make a crystal essence, but you must be sure it is not water-soluble and does not have any poisonous or metallic qualities. If in doubt, use clear quartz because it balances all the chakras.

To balance feminine problems associated with energy imbalances in Svadisthana, such as painful or irregular periods, a moonstone is ideal; it is also recommended for ridding the body of toxins and the emotional anxieties associated with 'mother issues'.

1 Wash and psychically cleanse the moonstone in clear water (see page 36).

2 Be clear about what you want to achieve, then ask for guidance from the crystal and follow what you intuit is right.

3 Place the crystal in a plain clear glass of distilled or pure spring water and cover it with a sheet of white paper or clear glass.

4 Leave in the sunshine (or daylight) for approximately three hours.

5 Remove the crystal and thank or bless it.

6 Slowly sip the water over the ourse of the day. It will have become encoded with beneficial vibrations from the crystal: this is an etheric imprint; nothing physical is transferred.

7 If you wish to keep the essence for a while, preserve it in pure brandy or vodka (50 per cent water: 50 per cent alcohol) and store it in a dark-coloured bottle away from sunlight and heat (a blue bottle is ideal). Stored bottles should not touch each other, and you should always keep them away from strong perfumes or chemical pollutants.

SACRAL CHAKRA MEDITATION

A good time for meditation is either following yoga practise or after crystal therapy. At such times, your body is already relaxed and ready for a session of focused concentration (see pages 22–23).

BEFORE YOU START

Choose a leisurely and relaxed time to meditate. If you like, create an atmosphere with oils, candles, or incense in the colour of the chakra. Sit or lie somewhere you won't be disturbed. You can pre-record the words of the meditation – dots indicate a pause.

1 As you lie motionless, become aware of change and movement that continues in your body ... your heartbeat ... blood flow around your body ... cellular activity that invisibly rejuvenates your whole being.

2 Focus on every breath. Each is a celebration of life ... nourishing you with everything you need for a healthy, enjoyable life.

3 Focus on the gentle movement of your abdomen rising and falling as you breathe. Imagine it filled with a warm, orange glow, representing joy and vitality, both of which are available to you in abundance ...

AFFIRMATIONS

• I am moving toward a time when I am totally happy and fulfilled. Life offers me everything I need for making that journey.

• I am worthy of love and sexual pleasure.

• I have a right to express my desires to myself and others.

• Who I am is good enough.

• My life is unfolding exactly as it should.

• I am prepared to honour my body and feel good about my sexuality.

4 Bring to mind a pleasurable experience from the past ... Recollect all the senses that will bring that moment back to life for you now ... Try to remember how you felt ... the colours around you ... textures ... shapes ... sounds ... smells ... tastes.

5 Shift that image to your abdomen so that the warm, orange glow suffuses it, magnifying the experience and making it even more satisfying and joyous ... Surrender your body entirely to the pleasures of that moment ... Tell yourself that this is something you deserve to experience every day of your life ... you can experience it again every time you put your mind to it ...

6 Know that your life can be a succession of wonderful, beneficial experiences if you choose it to be so ...

7 Come back slowly and gently to everyday awareness. Determine to look for the opportunities, the love, the joy, and the fun in all you do today. You deserve it.

DAILY QUESTIONS

- How much are you prepared to embrace change? Change one small thing today.

- How creative are you sexually? Discuss your sexual fantasies with your partner.

- What sacrifices do you make to suit others? Dysfunctional relationships are toxic to both. Try saying 'no' next time. Don't explain.

- Do you respect your female and male sides? It is alright to be soft one day, assertive the next. Different situations require different responses.

- Is it better to give than to receive? Accepting gifts, with pleasure, gives others something back. Do you deny them the joy of giving?

- Do you believe that for your desires to be met you first have to make a sacrifice? Focus on someone for whom life is sweet. Try mirroring them. Have you made a shift in your beliefs?

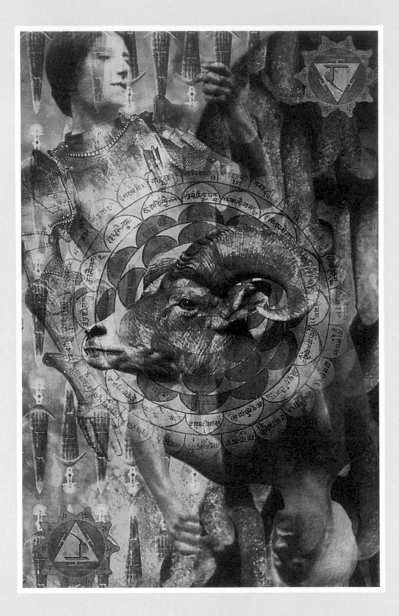

3
THE SOLAR PLEXUS CHAKRA: MANIPURA

The Solar Plexus Chakra, or Manipura, is also called, manipuraka, dashapatra, dashadala padma, dashapatrambuja, dashachchada, nabhi, nabhipadma and nabhipankaja. This chakra is traditionally located at the navel (hence the alternative name of the nabhi or navel chakra) because traditionalists believe the Solar Plexus refers to a distinct minor chakra

In the Indian Tantric tradition, Manipura – 'place of gems' or 'shining like a pearl' – has ten red petals, with a downward-pointing triangle, representing the element of Fire at the centre; however, in most modern chakra layouts it is placed at the Solar Plexus as a major chakra, with its ten petals shown in gold or yellow.

THE FUNCTIONS OF MANIPURA

Diverse cultures throughout the world have revered the energy symbolized by the Sun. Solar deities, usually masculine in nature, include Ra (Egyptian), Inti (Inca), Tonatiuih (Aztec), Ku-kuul-kaan (Maya), Mithras/Sol (European) and Vishnu/Indra (Hindu). Manipura's element, not surprisingly, is Fire. In Hindu tradition Agni is associated with fire and lightning together with the fearful goddess Kali, who often has

tongues of flame coming from her mouth. Think of Manipura as the Sun in your body. It draws in solar radiance as a type of prana and transduces it into a form that enables the flow of vital energies throughout the physical body to be regulated. It is a gathering point for lines of subtle energy, the nadis, which control all bodily functions, as well as being a powerful physical nerve plexus. The great Indian sage Patanjali says that through control of Manipura full mastery of the body is achieved.

Each petal represents an emotional aspect (see page 86). Together, they are to be overcome at this chakra level before proceeding to work on the Heart Chakra. It is important to note that the three major chakras below the heart are principally concerned with the physical body and the world we perceive with our senses, whereas those above the heart are of a more spiritual nature.

SOLAR PLEXUS CHAKRA CORRESPONDENCES

This chart for the Solar Plexus (Third) Chakra identifies the associations and symbolisms linked with this particular chakra. As such it provides a 'ready reference' of inspirations to use when choosing appropriate stones for crystal work. This chart will also help you with the various images you will need when composing your own meditations and visualizations. Incorporate as many of these symbols and themes as you feel is appropriate to your needs.

USING THE CHART

By re-acquainting yourself regularly with this chakra chart as a prelude to the entire section on the Solar Plexus Chakra, you will help focus your mind on its related issues. These include the development of your self-esteem as a precursor to achieving true personal power.

By strengthening and stimulating the Solar Plexus Chakra you will reach a state in which you can shake off the fears of rejection, criticism, and standing apart from the group,

You will be able to create your own, unique, identity – one that is founded on self-acceptance, self-respect, and the ability to take risks in the knowledge that you can handle any situation with which you are faced. This is true inner, personal power.

CHAKRA CHARACTERISTICS

See which of the following characteristics of excessive ('too open'), deficient ('blocked'), and balanced chakra energy you can relate to – and then determine (to take the necessary action, using the tools and techniques that follow.

- **Too open** (chakra spins too fast): angry, controlling, workaholic, judgemental and superior.

- **Blocked** (chakra spins sluggishly or not at all): overly concerned with what others think, fearful of being alone, insecure, needs reassurance.

- **Balanced** (chakra maintains equilibrium and spins at correct vibrational speed): respects self and others, has personal power, spontaneous, uninhibited.

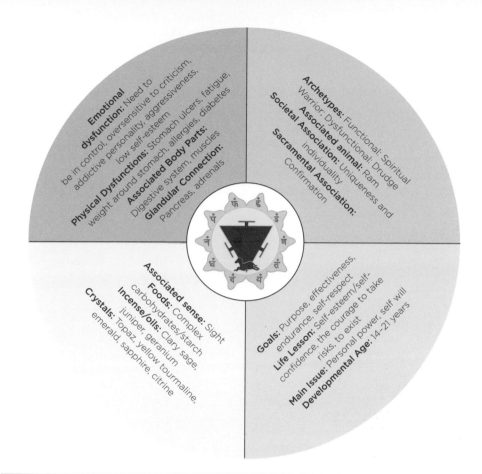

Emotional dysfunction: Need to be in control, oversensitive to criticism, addictive personality, aggressiveness, low self-esteem
Physical Dysfunctions: Stomach ulcers, fatigue, weight around stomach, allergies, diabetes
Associated Body Parts: Digestive system, muscles
Glandular Connection: Pancreas, adrenals

Archetypes: Functional: Spiritual Warrior; Dysfunctional: Drudge
Associated animal: Ram
Societal Association: Uniqueness and individuality
Sacramental Association: Confirmation

Associated sense: Sight
Foods: Complex carbohydrates/starch
Incense/oils: Clary sage, juniper, geranium
Crystals: Topaz, yellow tourmaline, emerald, sapphire, citrine

Goals: Purpose, effectiveness, endurance, self-respect
Life Lesson: Self-esteem/self-confidence, the courage to take risks, to exist
Main Issue: Personal power, self will
Developmental Age: 14–21 years

SOLAR PLEXUS CHAKRA	
Sanskrit name	Manipura
Meaning	Lustrous gem
Location	Between navel and base of sternum
Symbol	A ten-petalled lotus containing a downward pointing triangle (see page 86 for the yantra)
Associated colours	Yellow
Element	Fire
Ruling planet	Mars, Sun

SOLAR PLEXUS CHAKRA YANTRA

At the root of the navel is the shining lotus of ten petals, of the colour of heavily laden rain clouds. Meditate there on the region of Fire, triangular in form and shining like the rising sun. Outside of it are three Svastika marks, and within, the seed-mantra Ram. By meditating in this manner upon the navel lotus, the power to create and destroy the world is acquired.

— Sat Cakra Nirupana

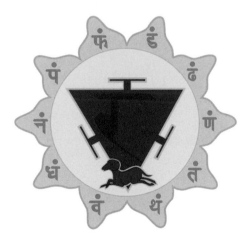

- **Colour:** The predominant colour of the Manipura yantra is a rich golden yellow. Sometimes the yantra is depicted as a greenish-blue colour.

- **Triangle:** At the centre of the Manipura yantra is a red, downward-pointing triangle. Each side of the triangle has a T-shaped projection. These projections symbolize movement

- **Ram:** At the base of the red, downward-pointing triangle is a ram. The ram represents the strength and courage of who we are in the world.

Some scholars believe that the ram in the yantra depicts the nature of a person dominated by the Manipura Chakra – strong in character, but has a tendency to charge head-first at times.

DESCRIPTION OF THE YANTRA

- **Number of petals:** The Manipura yantra has ten petals. Each of them represents a different emotion: spiritual ignorance; thirst; jealousy; treachery; shame; fear; disgust; delusion; foolishness; and sadness.

SOLAR PLEXUS CHAKRA ARCHETYPES

While the first two chakras have been concerned with our external relationships – the Root (First) Chakra with the group mind and the Sacral (Second) with specific relationships - the Solar Plexus (Third) Chakra is more internally focused: to our relationship with ourselves.

The ways in which we demonstrate our self-esteem and personal power is played out in the archetypes associated with this chakra – the Drudge and Spiritual Warrior.

THE DRUDGE

The Drudge continues the themes of lack of acknowledgement and reward seen in the Victim and Martyr. Drudges commonly regard being loveable in terms of what they do, not who they are and unconsciously look for relationships that reinforce that view. Hence the Drudge archetype can become involved with bullying, dominant partners.

Unfortunately the outside approval that Drudges desperately seek is not forthcoming, because this only happens when we learn to honour and value ourselves. Their inner chant of 'I am not worthy' needs to be erased in order for a true sense of self-worth to find its voice.

THE SPIRITUAL WARRIOR

The Spiritual Warrior is the hero or heroine who operates instinctively in their interactions with others, and always from a position of equality.

By meeting constant rejection or conflict, the Spiritual Warriors of myth and legend were forced to look inside themselves to make sense of those sets of circumstances and give them meaning. It is a truly powerful archetype when a spiritual philosophy of growth and development through facing life's obstacles is combined with acting with integrity, no matter how unpopular or inexplicable to others those actions may be.

The attributes of this functional archetype are the precursors to the power of love that is connected with the next chakra on our journey - the Heart. Because only by truly loving and honouring ourselves can we hope to act out of love and compassion toward others.

SOLAR PLEXUS CHAKRA AROMATHERAPY

The essential oil of sage (*Salvia officinalis*) is recommended for this chakra, but only for use in an oil diffuser (see page 30) because of its strong properties. Other plants, herbs and flower essences for Manipura include blackberry, buckthorn, loosestrife, mango and peppermint. If you use both the plant (herb) and the flower essence of the same type within an hour of each other, the effect is deepened for the body (herb) and the energy field (flower essence).

Blackberry assists the astral body; buckthorn strengthens the solar plexus; loosestrife promotes healing and flexibility and is sometimes used in athletes' massage cream; mango strengthens the Solar Plexus and Heart Chakras, and particularly the nadis (energy channels) in the chest; and peppermint calms down any digestive imbalances, especially those caused by stress held in Manipura.

SOLAR PLEXUS CHAKRA ESSENTIAL OILS

The main essential oils that have a sympathetic resonance with the Solar Plexus Chakra are:

- **Clary sage** This flowering plant is excellent for calming this chakra, although it should not be used if you have to drive afterwards, are taking alcohol or are pregnant (except during the early stages of labour, but only under medical supervision). Clary sage is the strongest relaxant known in aromatherapy and is capable of producing very euphoric states. It is anti-convulsive, anti-depressant, antiseptic, anti-spasmodic, emmenagogic and aphrodisiac.

- **Juniper** This oil comes from a small tree whose berries are crushed and the oil steam-distilled from them.

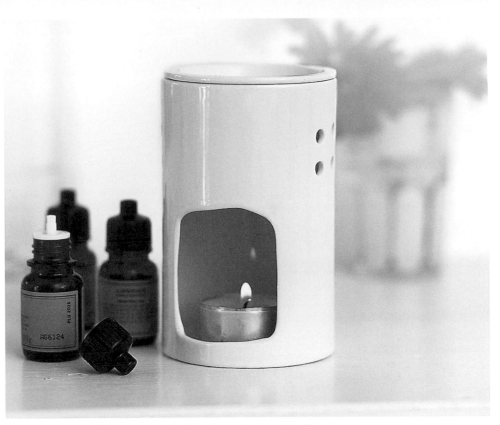

The oil diffuser holds water and a few drops of essential oil.

Jumiper oil is the main purifying essential oil used for massage and is ideal for clearing blockages from the Solar Plexus Chakra. Juniper really does clear out the body (rather like a tonic) and helps keep digestion running smoothly. It also happens to be the principal flavouring ingredient in gin, so perhaps the expression 'gin and tonic' was an apt one! Juniper is antiseptic, anti-spasmodic, emmenagogic and anti-toxic.

- **Geranium** The essential oil is made from the flowers, leaves and stalks. It is an adrenal-cortex stimulant and helps regulate hormone secretion throughout the endocrine system. An aromatherapist will also use it to detox the lymphatic system. It is an excellent oil to calm and balance Manipura, as it helps movement of pranic energy through the body. It is also anti-depressant, antiseptic, deodorant, diuretic and tonic, and excellent for treating PMS.

YOGA FOR THE SOLAR PLEXUS

Start your yoga session by balancing the chakras with a standing balanced asana (posture) such as Pranamasana (prayer pose). This is simply standing straight with the spine 'lifted', as if a cord is pulling it up from the crown of your head, and placing your hands together in the prayer position.

ACTIVE: COW

This pose stimulates the kidneys and pancreas, helping diabetic conditions, which are associated with imbalances in the Solar Plexus Chakra. The crossed and locked knee position and the arm position cause vital energy to be focused at this chakra.

The state of consciousness you are seeking at the Solar Plexus Chakra is manomaya kosha (the waking state), which is experienced through your intellectual mind. Use a visualization of a bright-yellow flaming Sun to help you, and draw breath into your body as a bright-yellow light.

1 Kneel down and sit on your heels, or sit with your knees crossed over one another (this is the advanced position).

2 Raise your left arm over your head, bending it at the elbow and turning it down your back. Bend your right arm up behind your back to catch your left hand with your right. Lock your fingers together. Hold the position for a while, then repeat on the opposite side.

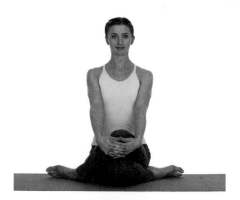
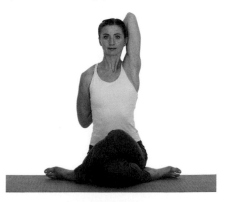

ACTIVE:
SITTING SPINAL TWIST

This asana benefits the kidneys and pancreas in a similar way to the Cow Pose. The intense twist of the spine works on the spinal nerves and, at a subtle level, improves energy flow through the ida and pingala nadis and the sushumna kundalini channel within the spine. However, the main focus is the massaging effect on the abdominal organs, which brings benefits to the Solar Plexus Chakra.

1 Sitting, bend your right knee and sit on the foot. Then bend your left knee and lift it over your right thigh, placing the foot flat on the floor.

2 Turn your body 90 degrees to the left and bring your right armpit over your left knee. Lock the arm over the knee, then move your left arm behind your waist, so that your left hand catches your right hand. Turn your neck to face left, looking over your left shoulder. Repeat on the opposite side.

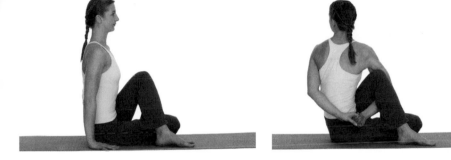

SIMPLE VERSION

1 Follow the steps above but turning to the other side.

2 Turning 90 degrees to the right, bring your left armpit over your right knee. Lock your arm over the knee.

3 Use your right arm to support and straighten your back. Repeat on the other side.

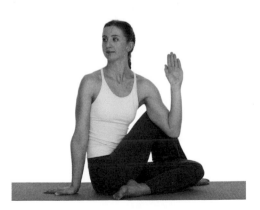

PASSIVE: CAMEL

The practice of this posture is recommended to keep your spine supple, work on the abdominal organs/muscles and the shoulder joints. During this intense stretch, focus on bringing a sparkling golden light into your Solar Plexus Chakra, where it will charge up and revitalize your whole body. If you have difficulty keeping your hips in line with your knees, place a cushion on top of your calves and tuck your toes under, to the ground, to raise your heels a bit. Only bend your back as far as feels comfortable.

1 Kneel on the floor with your buttocks raised off your feet. Gently lean backwards, placing your right hand on your right heel and your left hand on your left heel.

2 Push on your feet with your hands and, taking your head back, curve your spine upwards, pushing it up until your thighs are in line with your knees and the front of your body is straight. Relax into the position.

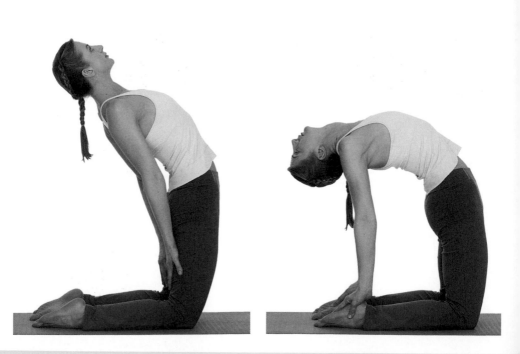

CRYSTALS TO ACTIVATE THE SOLAR PLEXUS CHAKRA

The gemstone crystals of topaz and yellow tourmaline are both recommended to activate Manipura.

TOPAZ

Topaz is obtainable in a number of colours, but for Manipura choose clear, bright yellow. A small raw crystal works fine; it is not necessary to have an expensive cut or polished one. Topaz assists in the realignment of energies, and helps to bring a golden radiance into the auric field. Traditionally, it is a crystal of love and fortune. With such clear energetic properties, it is an excellent aid to the whole body metabolism, but especially to the liver, gall bladder and digestive processes. It not only helps with digesting food, but also with the digestion of ideas at the mental level.

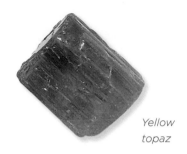

Yellow topaz

YELLOW TOURMALINE

Like other tourmalines, this one is very focused in a directional manner, and has the ability to balance the two sides of our brain and our male/female energies. When using it with the Solar Plexus Chakra, instead of placing it on the chakra, use the crystal to draw out or cut away blockages. This enables proper activation of Manipura, to benefit issues such as stress, intolerance, deep sadness, hopelessness, grief and conditions of 'dis-ease'.

Using crystals to boost energy flow

An excellent pick-me-up is to lie down and relax in the following way.

1 Obtain two clear quartz 'points' about 5 cm (2 in) long, plus one yellow stone or crystal: yellow topaz, yellow (not brown) citrine quartz or yellow tourmaline would be ideal. Cleanse them in the usual way (see page 36).

2 Ensure you are not going to be disturbed and switch off the telephone. If you wish, play some relaxing music to calm your mind.

3 Lie down, placing one quartz at your head and the other below your feet. It is vital that the point of each crystal faces in towards your body, not away from it.

4 Place your yellow crystal on your Manipura chakra. It is best if the stone is against your skin, but still works through clothing (especially white cotton clothing).

5 Take some deep breaths – relax – enjoy!

The effect of this session is to bring all the chakras into alignment through the central channel of the subtle-energy body. The yellow stone on Manipura helps it come into resonance with the others by clearing and purifying it.

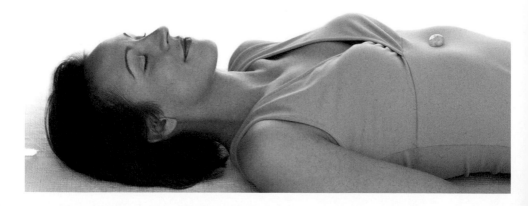

CRYSTALS TO CALM
THE SOLAR PLEXUS CHAKRA

With Manipura, a calming/slowing down of energies passing in and out through the chakra aids general well-being and improves concentration. This can enable us to study, work or meditate at deeper levels.

To discover if you are holding tension in your solar plexus, use your fingers to gently prod the area just below your sternum. Like as not you will find it sensitive or slightly sore to the touch. This indicates some stored tension. When it is seriously tense, the discomfort will extend from front to back and will cause back pain. When this condition worsens, it creates a horizontal band of tension, locking energy into the lower chakras. 'Dis-ease' of the physical body will quickly result from such blockages. Gemstone crystals to calm Manipura are emerald and sapphire.

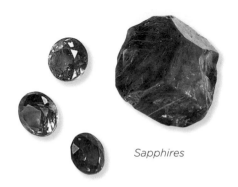

Sapphires

EMERALD

When used on Manipura, emerald will energetically calm imbalances associated with diabetes. It is also traditionally used for the liver, eyes and sinuses. It is said that if you always wear emerald as jewellery, you will experience negative emotions

SAPPHIRE

This crystal is gifted to us by Mother Nature in many colours. For the purpose of Manipura calming, use blue sapphire. In common with other blue precious stones, it opens you up to higher spiritual realms by calming the physical body. In particular it brings deep wisdom and serenity. It should be placed on the chakra position or held within the aura at a comfortable level. Energetically it regulates the endocrine system.

CRYSTALS TO BALANCE
THE SOLAR PLEXUS CHAKRA

When used on the Solar Plexus Chakra, yellow citrine helps individuals access their personal power. It enhances self-confidence and can help overcome an attraction to addictive substances, which is a common dysfunction of this chakra. On a physical level, yellow citrine benefits digestion.

CITRINE

Citrine is recommended as a good stone for general balancing of the Solar Plexus Chakra. It can be used in the form of a cluster, a point or a polished tumbled stone. For the exercise below, a selection of tumbled stones of a good clear yellow will be best and should not be too expensive. Try to avoid getting citrine that is a dark treacle-brown in colour, because it has been heat-treated and its power has changed.

Citrine has a sympathetic resonance with pranic energy coming from our Sun. It acts powerfully to cleanse, warm and energize. For this reason it balances our vibrational field so that we can walk consciously on Mother Earth, turning our eyes to the light that is manifesting through Father Sun. We have seen that Manipura symbolizes the Sun in our bodies. From ancient times people have revered the power within and beyond the Sun. We all need sunshine to keep our bodies healthy, and an excellent way to activate the Solar Plexus chakra is to 'breathe in' sunlight. Simply take deep breaths as you gaze at the Sun through half-closed eyes and visualize its energy focusing at the solar plexus and then filling your body. (Never be tempted to look directly at the Sun.)

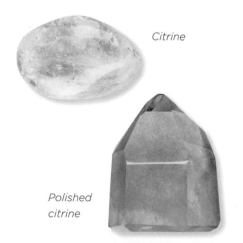

Citrine

*Polished
citrine*

Using citrine to balance yourself

Create a sacred space in your room; light a candle and some incense.

1 Lie on a blanket on the floor.

2 Place as many tumbled citrines as possible around the blanket in a circle (a minimum of six stones should suffice).

3 Lie down within the circle and allow yourself to relax.

4 If you wish, you can place another yellow stone on your Manipura Chakra point.

5 Affirm that you wish to balance your Solar Plexus Chakra, and ask for assistance from the hidden power of the citrine crystals.

6 Stay in the circle for up to 30 minutes.

7 Allow yourself to come back slowly to everyday awareness. Take your time.

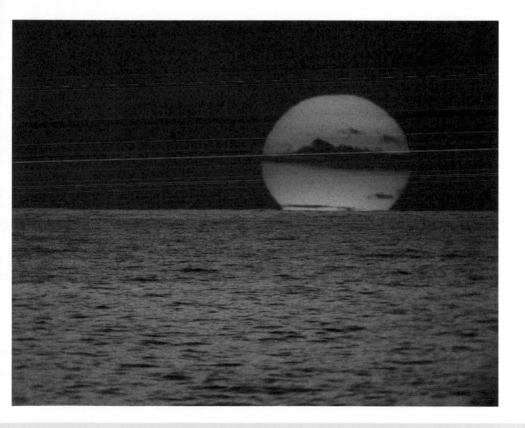

SOLAR PLEXUS CHAKRA MEDITATION

A good time for meditation is either following yoga practise or after crystal therapy. At such times, your body is already relaxed and ready for a session of focused concentration (see pages 22–23).

BEFORE YOU START

Choose a leisurely and relaxed time to meditate. If you like, create an atmosphere with oils, candles, or incense in the colour of the chakra. Sit or lie somewhere you won't be disturbed. You can pre-record the words of the meditation – dots indicate a pause.

1 You are on a path that winds up into the distance. The day is warm, with a gentle breeze, and you can feel the Sun on your back ... The air is perfumed with the scent of freshly mown grass and delicate flowers ...

2 As you gather pace, you feel the path incline steeply ... Ahead is a mountain and you slowly begin to ascend.

3 The sides of the mountain are steep and you must use all your intuition to select the safest path ...

4 Higher and higher you climb until you can see a plateau ...

There is a fire burning in the middle of this flat ground, its golden flames lapping the air ... You walk towards the fire.

AFFIRMATIONS

- I accept and value myself exactly as I am.

- I know I am becoming the best person I can be.

- I determine to treat myself with honour and respect.

- My personal power is becoming stronger each day.

- I am my own person. I choose how to think and behave.

- I deserve all the love, respect, joy, and prosperity that comes to me. I am open to receiving all life's good things.

5 By the fire is a pen and paper ... Stop, pick them up and think about a person(s) to whom you have relinquished personal power ...

6 Write the name(s) on the paper and hold it out to the flame ... Watch the fire eat the paper until it is utterly destroyed ...

7 Bathe yourself in the warmth of the fire; feel its heat regenerate your Solar Plexus, strengthening it ... Connect with the power of your Solar Plexus ... Know that you are a spiritual warrior and that you have the inner resources to help you overcome all life's challenges ...

8 Revel in this moment of personal power and notice how it feels ... tune in to the signals that your body gives you so that you will recognize them again ...

9 Now it's time to turn away from the flame, climb down from the top of the mountain and find the safest path down ... You are the same, but different ...

10 Your power store is now stronger than it was and will become more so every time you visit the flame on the mountain top ... And you can do so any time you choose. Return to your everyday surroundings.

DAILY QUESTIONS

- What risks can you take to strengthen your personal power base? Consider confronting your fears about a particular person. How could you equalize your relationship with him/her?

- Have you recently acted subserviently? Did you gain anything? How can you prevent this happening again? Visualize a more empowering outcome.

- Who do you admire who 'owns' themselves? How do they demonstrate personal power? How can you emulate them? If you admire a public figure, learn about them. When you are faced with a challenging decision, imagine what choice they would make.

- How do you use your anger? Controlled anger is a healthy expression of personal power. Practise giving vent to anger by punching a cushion or pillow.

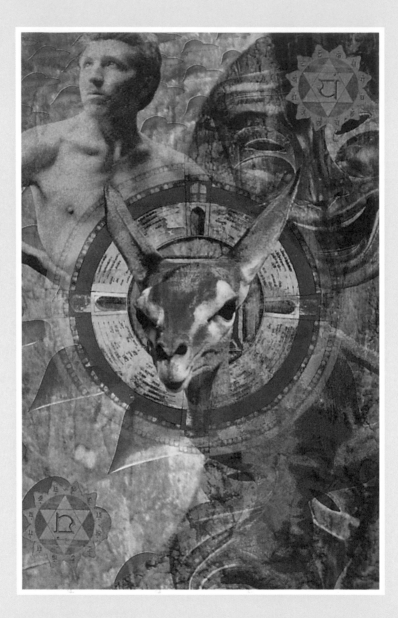

4 THE HEART CHAKRA: ANAHATA

The Heart Chakra or Anahata is also known as anahata-puri, padma-sundara, dwadasha, dwadashadala, suryasangkhyadala, hrit padma, hridaya chakra, dwadashara chakra and by various other names.

In Tantric teachings, Anahata (meaning 'unstruck note') has 12 red or white petals, while the central part is a smoky-blue/black colour symbolizing the element of Air. Anahata is positioned in the centre of the chest and is connected to the Thymus Chakra.

THE FUNCTIONS OF ANAHATA

Each of the 12 petals of Anahata represents a different human trait (see page 104). The chakra is associated with the element (or tattwa) of Air, and is the seat of the Divine Soul or Higher Self, the Jivatman, represented by the image of a motionless golden lamp-flame.

Anahata is linked to the ages of 22 to 28, when we are often forming deep relationships, hopefully based on reciprocal love. But the Heart Chakra is not primarily about falling in love; it is not a sentimental kind of love. Instead its fire is fuelled by the love of creation – the same love that causes us to delight in the feel of soft rain on our skin or the heady perfume of a sweet-scented flower.

Anahata is at the centre of our luminous auric body. The colour of light to balance it is a bright grass-green, and quite commonly the 12 petals are shown in this colour. Anahata is the midpoint in the seven chakras and rests at the midpoint in the body. For these reasons, it is considered to be the gateway to higher consciousness.

In Tibetan Buddhism, the Heart Chakra is depicted as a white, eight-petalled heart centre, the meeting place of the 'Red and White Drops', seat of the 'Very Subtle Mind' and 'Very Subtle Wind', which are immortal and pass from one lifetime to the next.

In Taoism, this chakra is the House of Fire. It is located at the top of the central 'Thrusting Channel', and is the counterbalance to the Lower Tan Tien, or House of Water.

HEART CHAKRA CORRESPONDENCES

The chart for the Heart (Fourth) Chakra identifies all the associations and symbolisms linked with this particular chakra. As such it provides a 'ready reference' of inspirations to use when you carry out practical exercises such as choosing appropriate stones for crystal work.

USING THE CHART

The chart will also help you with the various images you will need when composing your own meditations and visualizations. Incorporate as many of these symbols and themes as you feel is appropriate to your needs.

By reaquainting yourself regularly with this chakra as a prelude to the entire section on the Heart Chakra, you will help keep your mind focused on related issues, including an awareness of the opportunities for growth and development that come from forming loving relationships with others. Mastering the Heart Chakra helps us to enhance our emotional development and recognize the potency of that powerful energy we call 'love'.

CHAKRA CHARACTERISTICS

See which of the following characteristics of excessive ('too open'), deficient ('blocked'), and balanced chakra energy you can relate to - and then determine (should you choose) to take the necessary action, using the tools and techniques outlined on the following pages in this chapter.

- **Too open** (chakra spins too fast): possessive, loves conditionally, witholds emotionally 'to punish', overly dramatic.

- **Blocked** (chakra spins sluggishly or not at all): fears rejection, loves too much, feels unworthy to receive love, self-pitying.

- **Balanced** (chakra maintains equilibrium and spins at correct vibrational speed): compassionate, loves unconditionally, nurturing, desires spiritual experience in lovemaking.

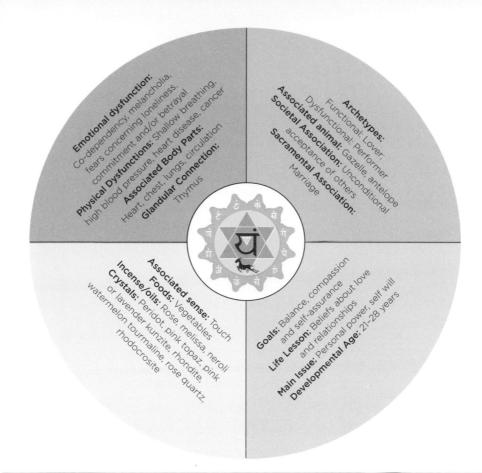

Archetypes:
Functional: Lover.
Dysfunctional: Performer
Associated animal: Gazelle, antelope
Societal Association: Unconditional
acceptance of others
Sacramental Association:
Marriage

Emotional dysfunction:
Co-dependency, melancholia,
fears concerning loneliness,
commitment and/or betrayal
Physical Dysfunctions: Shallow breathing,
high blood pressure, heart disease, cancer
Associated Body Parts:
Heart, chest, lungs, circulation
Glandular Connection:
Thymus

Associated sense: Touch
Associated Foods: Vegetables
Incense/oils: Rose, melissa, neroli
Crystals: Peridot, pink topaz, pink
or lavender kunzite, rhondite,
watermelon tourmaline, rose quartz,
rhodocrosite

Goals: Balance, compassion
and self-assurance
Life Lesson: Beliefs about love
and relationships
Main Issue: Personal power, self will
Developmental Age: 21–28 years

HEART CHAKRA	
Sanskrit name	Anahata
Meaning	Sound that is made without any two things striking; unstruck
Location	Centre of chest
Symbol	Lotus of 12 petals, containing two intersecting circles that make up a six-pointed star (see page 104 for the yantra).
Associated colours	Green, pink
Element	Air
Ruling planet	Venus

HEART CHAKRA YANTRA

In the heart is the charming lotus of the colour of the Bandhuka flower. It is like Kalpa-taru, the celestial wishing tree, bestowing even more than desire.

— Sat Cakra Nirupana

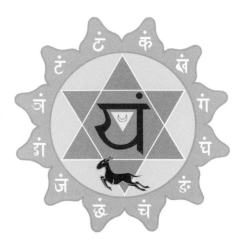

DESCRIPTION OF THE YANTRA

- **Number of petals:** The Anahata yantra has twelve petals, each one representing a different human trait: lustfulness; fraudulence; indecision; repentance; hope; anxiety; longing; impartiality; arrogance; incompetence; discrimination; an attitude of defiance.

- **Colour:** Green or vermilion.

- **Element:** Air.

- **Star:** At the centre of the Anahata yantra are two triangles superimposed on each other to form a star shape. This represents balance and harmony.

- **Golden triangle:** At the centre of the star sits a downward-pointing triangle. This indicates the Divine light that can be revealed when this chakra is fully opened.

- **Crescent moon:** A crescent moon that sits at the centre of the golden triangle represents the granthis of Vishnu, the psychic blocks that must be dissolved in order to achieve true enlightenment.

- **Antelope or deer:** At the base of the Anahata yantra, the depiction of an antelope or deer refers to the lightness and speed of the Air element. According to legend, Avayu, the Vedic god of the winds, rode a deer.

HEART CHAKRA ARCHETYPES

The Heart (Fourth) Chakra further develops the internal focus that started with the lower chakras and is concerned with balancing the love of others and the love of ourselves. This central chakra is the passage through which we move from the lower to the higher centres, shifting us from the realm of basic needs into the realm of blessings. Our challenge is to pass the tests of unconditional love, compassion, and forgiveness with which we are challenged daily, in order to move on to the higher centres.

As we make our journey toward the Higher Self our relationships painfully expose us to how little we love ourselves. When we strip away the thin veneer that covers lack of self-intimacy and fill it energetically with joy, peace, and self-acceptance, we start to build the solid foundation upon which unconditional love flourishes. Those who dismiss or shun intimacy demonstrate their fear of looking inward. They neglect the opportunities that relationships offer for self-knowledge – acknowledging and loving our dark side as well as the parts we admire. This is the basis of unconditional love. The archetypes associated with the Heart Chakra are the Performer and the Lover.

THE PERFORMER

Performers mask personal wounds by playing at being 'in love'; a very different experience to truly loving someone. Their way is a theoretical, cerebral, activity, without putting heart and soul into the relationship.

THE LOVER

True Lovers have the capacity to love themselves unconditionally. Because they don't need other people to buoy them up, they freely open their hearts and share self-acceptance with others. These generous, free-spirited, individuals offer themselves wholeheartedly to others because they know that the core of their being is secure. Being in touch with their emotions, they take a lighter approach to relationships, in the certain knowledge that the forgiveness and compassion, which their dysfunctional counterparts look to others to provide, is available to them internally at any time.

HEART CHAKRA AROMATHERAPY

The scents of plants, trees and herbs benefit us in many ways: the scent exuding from the bark of birch enables us to find inner peace, while chamomile leaves and flowers give off a scent that has a strongly sedative effect, which opens the Heart Chakra and works on our emotional levels.

Olive leaf taken as a herb tincture strengthens the immune system, and pear-flower essence is recommended for inspiring musicians. Strawberry and pomegranate, either eaten as fruits or taken as flower essences strengthen the Heart Chakra. Strong-smelling thyme, as a herb or flower essence, works on the physical heart/thymus connections.

HEART CHAKRA ESSENTIAL OILS

The main essential oils that have a sympathetic resonance with the Heart Chakra are:

• **Rose** This oil moves the energy of passion to that of unconditional love. When used with the energies of Anahata, it is also valuable as an anti-depressant following bereavement or the breakdown of a relationship with a loved one. It is antiseptic, emmenagogic, hepatic, sedative and uterine.

• **Melissa** This makes a good alternative to rose for massage to benefit the physical and etheric heart, but take care when using it on those with sensitive skin. It has a slightly lemony perfume and enhances rose, lavender and geranium essential oils. Melissa is recommended for shock or grief and lowers high blood pressure. It has a sedative effect and strengthens Anahata. It is expensive and needs to be used sparingly. The wise Greek healer Paracelsus called melissa 'the elixir of life'. It is anti-depressant, antiseptic, anti-spasmodic, anti-viral, febrifuge, nervine and sedative.

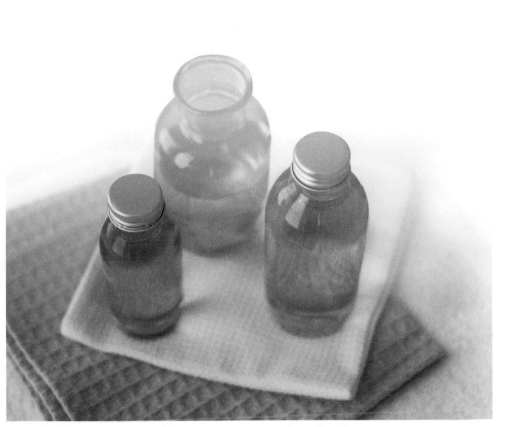

Aromatherapy oils, used in a diffuser or massage, can benefit us in many ways.

- **Neroli** This is the number-one oil for treating stress or shock. It is made from the blossom of the bitter orange tree, has an extremely strong perfume and blends well with other oils. It is very beneficial for the skin, especially for rejuvenating dry or ageing skin. However, as a Heart Chakra oil, it is also superb, since it acts as an anti-depressant, a sedative and an aphrodisiac.

MASSAGE AND VAPORIZATION

A massage by a trained aromatherapist using a blend that includes any of the oils opposite, will be a really pleasurable experience. If you are unable to have a massage, perhaps the next best thing is to enjoy the perfumes and therapeutic properties of these oils, by using them in a bath or an oil diffuser (see page 30).

YOGA FOR THE HEART CHAKRA

Start your yoga session by balancing the chakras with a standing balanced asana (posture) such as Pranamasana (prayer pose). This is simply standing straight with the spine 'lifted', as if a cord is pulling it up from the crown of your head, and placing your hands together in the prayer position.

ACTIVE: COBRA

Physically, the Cobra works powerfully on the spine. The position should never be forced – only extend it within your own comfortable range. This asana opens and allows the beautiful symbolic lotus at the Heart Chakra to 'flower'. Visualize the flower opening, revealing golden stamens in the centre like precious jewels. The state of consciousness you are seeking at the Heart Chakra is visnanamaya (awareness), your own personal experience of your wisdom body.

1 Lie flat on the floor, with your chin resting down. Place your hands flat on the floor under your shoulders, with your fingers pointing forwards.

2 Gently raise your body to a comfortable height as you curve your back backwards. Keep your pubis in contact with the floor – do not lift your body right off the floor. Your arms do not have to be fully extended; you may bend your elbows. Flexibility of your spine will develop with practice.

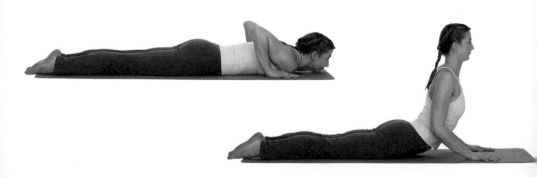

PASSIVE: HEAD-TO-KNEE FORWARD BEND

This asana stretches the backs of the leg muscles and loosens the hip joints, toning the abdominal organs and stretching the spine throughout its entire length. If you find sitting-forward bends difficult because your spine and hips are not very flexible, sit with your tailbone on the edge of a hard cushion to improve your flexibility from the hip joint. While bending forwards, always endeavour to flatten your back as much as possible – this has the effect of opening the Heart Chakra. Remember that chakras open to the front and back (with the exception of the Root and Crown Chakras), so focus on light coming into the centre middle of your back. Use the yantra as a focus, or the colour of a bright fresh green being drawn into your lungs and heart. This brings balance and harmony into the Heart Chakra as you relax into the posture. Only once you are extremely supple will you achieve the asana shown in step 2.

1 Sit with both legs flat on the floor in front of you. Bend your right knee and move it to the right, tucking your right heel close to the crotch area. Catch your left big toe with both hands.

2 Lift your head, then on an out-breath bend forwards over your left leg, to bring your face as close to your left knee as possible. Repeat with the opposite leg.

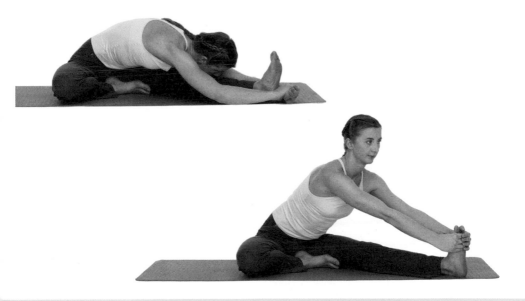

PASSIVE: FISH

This asana strengthens the chest, neck and spine, as well as the respiratory system, and bending the body upwards in this way benefits Anahata. There are two versions with different degrees of difficulty.

1 Easy posture: lie on the floor with your legs stretched straight out. Place your hands or elbows on the floor to support you, then arch your back and place the top of your head gently on the floor, keeping your chest raised.

2 Advanced posture: sit with your legs crossed in a full lotus position and, on an exhalation, lie backwards, supporting yourself on your elbows, until the top of your head just rests on the floor. Bring your hands to catch your toes.

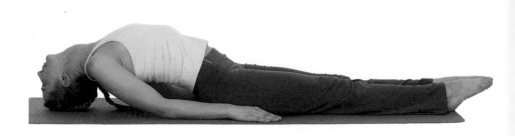

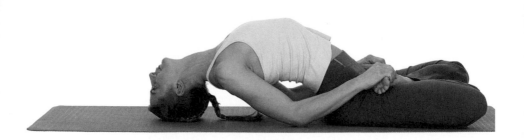

CRYSTALS TO ACTIVATE THE HEART CHAKRA

When we talk of activating a chakra, we imply that it is lacking in energetic flow. However, you need to ascertain if this really is the case, by a diagnostic method; or, if you prefer, simply use one of the balancing crystals shown on the following pages. The main crystal used to activate Anahata is peridot.

PERIDOT

Nature has given us the gift of this high-energy gemstone, which is also known by crystal therapists as chrysolite and olivine. Its colours range from a brownish-green to a bright clear green, and it is the latter colour that is used to activate the Heart Chakra.

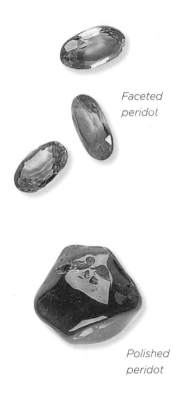

Faceted peridot

Peridot activates Anahata in many diverse ways: first, it is regarded as a cleansing stone, capable of clearing out toxins from the aura and physical body. Then, on a psychological level, it assists negative emotions that may originate from the heart, such as jealousy, envy, hate and anger, and helps move these emotions out through the chakra. It can therefore be seen as 'the stone of relationships' – easing away negative emotions that hold us back from truly loving, and replacing them with compassion, love and calmness.

Polished peridot

Using peridot to boost your energy vibrations

On a physical level peridot can be useful in assisting with the energetic vibrations of the heart and lungs.

One way to use peridot is to make a crystal essence using the indirect method (see page 39). Essentially, this involves leaving a cleansed crystal in a glass of pure spring water overnight (preferably in moonlight) and then slowly sip the water in the morning – being careful to remove the small crystal first!

When using any crystal healing method, remember that 'dis-ease' has probably taken a long time to lodge itself in the physical body, having passed through all the levels of the aura to get there. You need, therefore, consciously to ease the dis-ease out again, dissolving any patterns or imprints that predispose you to it. This usually requires time and dedication. And of course you must follow any medical advice, and create the optimum conditions for your return to health, such as nutritious food, relaxation and a healthy lifestyle.

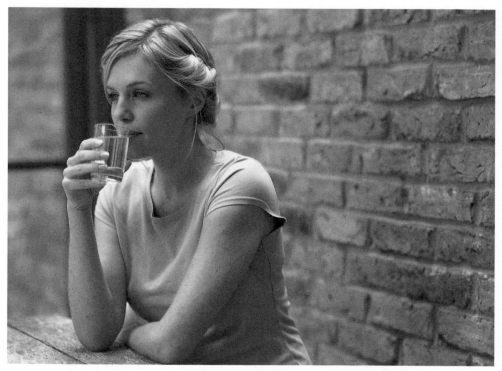

Sipping peridot-infused spring water can assist the vibrations of energy in the heart.

CRYSTALS TO CALM THE HEART CHAKRA

The most effective crystals for calming the energies of the Heart Chakra are blue sapphire (see page 95), pink topaz, pink kunzite and rhodonite.

PINK TOPAZ

This is a rare gemstone with a special correspondence to our heart and that of Mother Earth. In Native American traditions, crystals – sometimes referred to as 'frozen light' – are seen as the precious endocrine glands of Mother Earth's body. Therefore, when using pink topaz, we create an immediate synergy with the Thymus Chakra that is closely associated with the heart. Pink topaz disperses old patterns of 'dis-ease' that are held in the auric field relating to the heart.

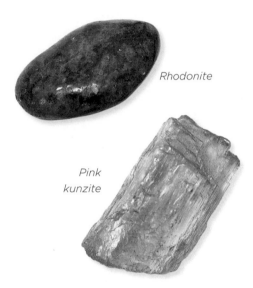

Rhodonite

Pink kunzite

PINK OR LAVENDER KUNZITE

This is an excellent crystal to use at the Heart Chakra. Pink and lavender kunzite especially help to heal the pain of broken relationships or loss through death. Kunzite is always calming to the Heart Chakra, by bringing into the auric field increased levels of compassion. It is used to help lift depression arising from emotional turbulence, and to calm panic attacks.

RHODONITE

Rhodonite is used to clear unwanted energies and to calm, and it is recommended that you use it for this purpose before placing any other crystal on the Heart Chakra. Because of its iron content (the black streaks), it grounds you and enables deeper work to take place towards the ideal of unconditional love. You can then bring balance to Anahata.

CRYSTALS TO BALANCE THE HEART CHAKRA

Watermelon tourmaline, green aventurine, rose quartz, rhodonite (see page 113) and rhodocrosite may all be used to balance Anahata. They are best used as small, tumble-polished stones, with the exception of watermelon tourmaline, which is usually cut in 'slices' to show off its naturally occurring pink heart in the midst of the green crystal.

WATERMELON TOURMALINE

This is the first choice to use for balancing the Heart Chakra. It is said to be the 'superactivator' of the Heart Chakra, allowing this area to become connected with the Higher Self. The green part brings life-force energy into the body, while the pink soothes and harmonizes. Watermelon tourmaline helps to reconcile opposites and confusion about sexual roles. It can teach us to be self-contained, integrated and in loving harmony with all the different aspects of ourselves.

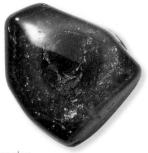

Watermelon tourmaline

RHODOCROSITE

This is a good energy conductor, as it has a high copper content. It integrates physical, mental and emotional aspects at the heart level. It is an ideal crystal to give back to the Earth as an offering, if you are in a special place.

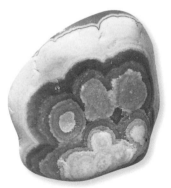

Rhodocrosite

ROSE QUARTZ

This stone will bring you both friendship and love. It is an ideal crystal to give a friend, as it has gentle, caring energies. In meditation it will take you through opening the different levels of the Heart Chakra and find ways to connect you with your inner cosmic child. In the physical body, rose quartz can aid sexual and emotional imbalance and increase fertility. You can hold a rose quartz in each hand while you meditate.

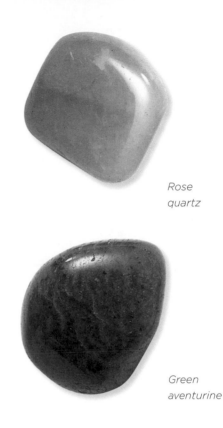

Rose quartz

Green aventurine

GREEN AVENTURINE

This crystal both calms Anahata and balances the energies of the heart and lungs. It is a sparkly green quartz with good all-round healing abilities. To balance your whole body, you should try the following exercise.

Using green aventurine to balance heart energies

1 Place a square of bright green cloth on the floor (silk is best, but cotton will do – do not use artificial fibres).

2 Arrange as many tumbled green aventurine stones as you can find in a perfect circle around the cloth. (Cleanse all the crystals both before and after use, see page 36.)

3 Next, lie down on your back on the cloth, with your head to the north, and so that it is centred within your circle of stones.

4 In the centre of your chest place another aventurine and four quartz points, equally spaced in the north, south, east and west directions, with the points facing inwards towards the aventurine.

5 Relax for about half an hour.

HEART CHAKRA MEDITATION

A good time for meditation is either following yoga practise or after crystal therapy. At such times, your body is already relaxed and ready for a session of focused concentration (see pages 22–23).

BEFORE YOU START

Choose a leisurely and relaxed time to meditate. If you like, create an atmosphere with oils, candles, or incense in the colour of the chakra. Sit or lie somewhere you won't be disturbed. You can pre-record the words of the meditation – dots indicate a pause.

1 You are beginning a journey to the Heart Chakra ... Are you nervous, excited, pained? Acknowledge these feelings, but don't dwell on them ... Know that you are safe, loved ...

2 See yourself on a red pathway. Feel firm earth beneath your feet ... Notice the road changing to sandy orange, then rippling beneath your feet like water. Your feet seem lighter and help you move on ...

3 The road changes again, to a rich golden yellow ... Feel its warmth penetrate your feet, warming your entire being ... Everything is bathed in golden sunlight ...

AFFIRMATIONS

- I send love to everyone I know; all hearts are open to receive my love.

- I accept that pain is an essential part of my growth and development.

- I love myself for who I am and the potential within me.

- All past hurt I release into the hands of love.

- I am grateful for all the love that is in my life.

- Other people deserve my compassion.

- The love I feel for myself and others is unconditional.

- Love will set me free.

4 Look ahead. The road has become green and leads to a pink castle ... As you take this green pathway it falls away beneath you, as if you're walking on air ... You are now at the entrance of the pink castle.

5 Feel the heavy door swing open into a vast pink hall ... On a plinth lies your heart. How does it look? Is it frozen in a block of ice? Or encased in chains? Or is it haemorrhaging energy from being too open to others ... Consider its state ... Don't judge what you see - you're here to heal it ...

6 Have the appropriate remedy available to you. Take a pick and chip away at the ice, breathing warm air to melt it faster ... Unlock the chains with a key from your pocket ...

7 Place your hands lovingly on any scars and send Universal Love to your heart to dissolve them ...

8 How does your heart respond to this attention? ... Be aware of a connection between what is in your mind's eye and what is going on in your body ... Enjoy these moments ...

9 Caress your heart and send it limitless Universal Love, knowing that the more it receives the more love will be available to others.

DAILY QUESTIONS

- Do you respond to others through the mind and intellect rather than the Heart? Tune in to your Heart's message. Focus on what you truly feel, without judging. The Heart has the answers.

- How much do you feel connected with others? Try going out and smiling at people. You'll be surprised how many smile back.

- Are you hard on yourself for 'failing'? This chakra is about balance - not just with others but with yourself.

- Learn to detach from your feelings. When your heart is full of pain, acknowledge that it represents another lesson. Rejoice and move on.

- Are you compassionate, or do you judge others? Everyone's reality is different. Know that no-one can hurt you - it's how you react to what they do to you that is the cause of your pain.

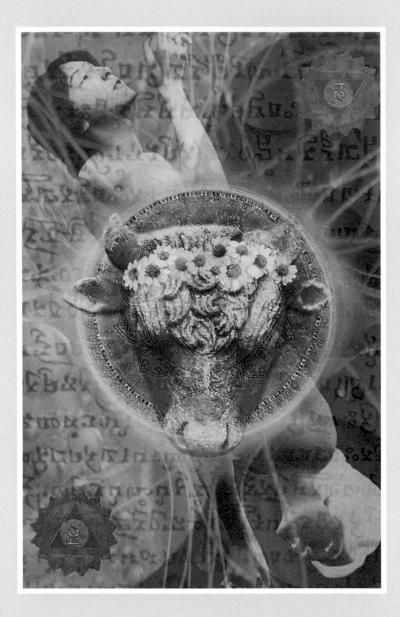

5 THE THROAT CHAKRA: VISHUDDA

The Throat Chakra or Vishuddha is known as kantha, kanthadesha, kanthapadma, kanthapankaja, shodasha, kanthambhoja, shodasha-dala, akasha, nirmala-padma, shodashara, dwyashtapatrambuja and by other names. The element associated with this chakra is ether/akasha, through which are transmitted the subtle vibrations of mantras, as used in Laya yoga.

Vishuddha means 'to purify'. In Tantric yoga, this chakra has 16 smoke-coloured petals, each linked with one of the Sanskrit vowels, a mantra or a musical tone. The central chakra region is white, transparent, smoke or sky-blue in colour, although modern interpretations of the Throat Chakra usually show the 16 petals in a turquoise colour.

THE FUNCTIONS OF VISHUDDHA

Vishuddha is regarded as an important 'bridge' from the heart, in the raising of consciousness through the sequential activation of the chakras from the root to the crown of the head. In a sense Vishuddha really is a bridge, because it takes us from one side of the 'river of life' – our body – to the other side, into spiritual realms. Of the 16 petals, the first represents Pranava (the mantra OM/AUM); the next seven represent mantras; and the last eight are associated with nectar and seven musical tones.

It is the place from where we can speak or sing our love: for our partner, our world, our god/s, our goddess. Conversely we can use our voice to hurt or slander, speaking bitter words that destroy and turn the energies of this chakra inwards. Vishuddha will not continue to receive sustenance from the sacred ether unless we can speak and sing good words.

Energy imbalances in Vishuddha manifest as ear, nose, throat and respiratory problems in the physical body. So if there is discomfort or 'dis-ease' in these areas, the Throat Chakra will be the first one to give healing to. As it comes into balance, we learn to feel truly that we are 'in our body' and can express the creative and life-affirming aspects of ourselves.

THROAT CHAKRA CORRESPONDENCES

This chart for the Throat (Fifth) Chakra identifies all the associations and symbolisms linked with this particular chakra. As such it provides a 'ready reference' of inspirations to use when you carry out practical exercises such as choosing appropriate stones for crystal work.

USING THE CHART

This chart will also help you with the various images you will need when composing your meditations and visualizations. Incorporate as many of these symbols and themes as you feel is appropriate to your needs.

By reacquainting yourself regularly with this chakra chart as a prelude to the section on the Throat Chakra, you will help to keep your mind focused on related issues, including the importance of expressing your emotions and communicating your truth to yourself and others.

Mastering the Throat Chakra helps us grasp the importance of purifying ourselves by honestly recognizing how we feel and having the confidence to communicate those emotions to others.

CHAKRA CHARACTERISTICS

See which of the following characteristics of excessive ('too open'), deficient ('blocked'), and balanced chakra energy you can relate to - and then determine (should you choose) to take the necessary action, using the tools and techniques outlined in this chapter.

- **Too open** (chakra spins too fast): over-talkative, dogmatic, self-righteous, arrogant.

- **Blocked** (chakra spins sluggishly or not at all): holds back from self-expression, unreliable, holds inconsistent views.

- **Balanced** (chakra maintains equilibrium and spins at correct vibrational speed): good communicator, contented, finds it easy to meditate, artistically inspired.

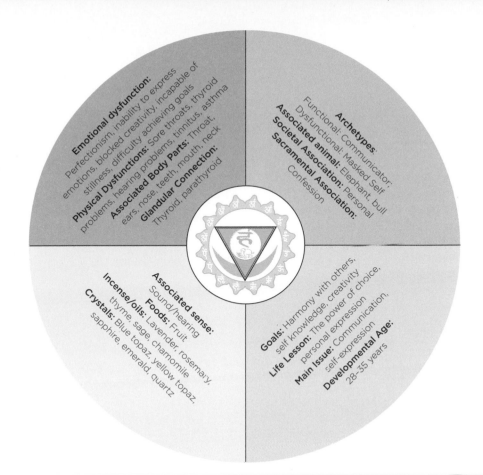

Emotional dysfunction: Perfectionism, inability to express emotions, blocked creativity, incapable of stillness, difficulty achieving goals
Physical Dysfunctions: Sore throats, thyroid problems, hearing problems, tinnitus, asthma
Associated Body Parts: Throat, ears, nose, teeth, mouth, neck
Glandular Connection: Thyroid, parathyroid

Archetypes: Functional: Communicator; Dysfunctional: Masked Self
Associated animal: Elephant, bull
Societal Association: Personal
Sacramental Association: Confession

Associated sense: Sound/hearing
Foods: Fruit
Incense/oils: Lavender, rosemary, thyme, sage, chamomile
Crystals: Blue topaz, yellow topaz, sapphire, emerald, quartz

Goals: Harmony with others, self knowledge, creativity
Life Lesson: The power of choice, personal expression
Main Issue: Communication, self-expression
Developmental Age: 28–35 years

THROAT CHAKRA	
Sanskrit name	Vishudda
Meaning	Purification
Location	Centrally, at the base of the neck
Symbol	Lotus of 16 petals, containing a downward-pointing triangle (see page 122 for the yantra)
Associated colour	Blue
Element	Ether
Ruling planet	Mercury

THROAT CHAKRA YANTRA

In the throat is the Lotus called Vishuddha, which is pure. This is the gateway of great liberation for him who desires the wealth of Yoga and whose senses are pure and controlled. He sees past, present and future and becomes the benefactor of all, free from disease and sorrow and long-lived.

— Sat Cakra Nirupana

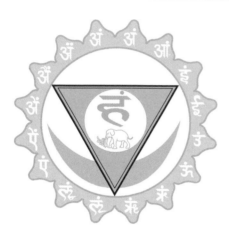

DESCRIPTION OF THE YANTRA

- **Number of petals:** The Vishuddha yantra as a total of 16 petals. Each of them represents either a Sanskrit vowel, a musical note or a mantra.

- **Colour:** The Vishuddha yantra is either blue or blue-grey.

- **Triangle:** Within the white circle sits a yellow, downward-pointing triangle. This is known as an akasamandala.

- **Silver crescent:** Behind the downward-pointing triangle, at the base of the yantra, sits a silver crecscent moon. This is the symbol of the cosmic sound, nadam, which represents purity.

- **White circle:** Within the yellow, downward-pointing triangle there is a white circle. This represents the full Moon, our psychic powers and the element Ether.

- **White elephant:** At the centre of the Vishuddha yantra is a white elephant, the animal guardian, Alravata, who carries the sound mantra. Airvata is associated with the god Indra. He has no restraining collar – he is servitude, transformed into service.

HEART CHAKRA ARCHETYPES

The next time you meet someone who appears to have trouble expressing themselves, see if their chin is held down on the chest, hiding the throat area in a childlike manner. This shows that this person has a vulnerability in the Throat (Fifth) Chakra.

Such people have frequently to clear the throat because esoterically it is being choked by the truths they are having to swallow. They may attempt to contribute to group discussions, but because of inarticulateness or lack of enthusiasm they are frequently not 'heard'. These are clues to a dysfunctional Throat Chakra.

THE MASKED SELF

In its extreme form the negative archetype associated with the Throat Chakra is the Masked Self. Here we have someone incapable of openly and honestly expressing feelings. They may wish to refuse an unreasonable (or reasonable) request, but say 'yes' anyway. Anger and frustration then builds up, further blocking the Throat Chakra, which may manifest itself physically as sore throat, glandular fever, stiff neck, and thyroid problems. The silence is not of lack of communication but lack of truthful expression.

THE COMMUNICATOR

Communicators often have wonderful speaking voices that others delight in listening to. They may have jobs in the areas of public speaking, teaching, broadcasting and various therapies. That is not to say that all who work in these fields are true Communicators – but the ones who excel undoubtedly do so because they express themselves with amazing clarity. It is the congruence that listeners sense between their self-expression and sincerity of the inner Self that makes Communicators so compelling.

Communicators recognize their right to express their hurt or anger, but do so in such a way that it doesn't diminish the other person. They integrate both heart and mind in their communications with others. They also recognize the power of the spoken and written word and, by taking responsibility for their feelings, do not abuse them.

THROAT CHAKRA AROMATHERAPY

Of the many plants, herbs and flower essences suitable for use on Vishuddha, chickweed and cleavers are best used as the dried or fresh herb or in tinctures – they are generally cleansing to the body.

Grapefruit as an extract helps weight loss, strengthens the immune system and is a cleansing tonic after illness. Magnolia-bark tea can assist meditation on past lives, as well as harmonizing the Heart and Throat Chakras. Marshmallow softens negative traits associated with Vishuddha. And willow flower enables the release of old pains and sadness.

THROAT CHAKRA ESSENTIAL OILS

The main essential oils that have a sympathetic resonance with Vishuddha are:

• **Lavender** This is one of the safest and most versatile essential oils. It is excellent in the bath (use 5 drops), in a vaporizer (burner), or as 2 drops on a handkerchief. It is the number-one choice in a home first-aid kit for insect bites, migraine, nausea, minor burns, stings, sunburn, small cuts, chilblains, eczema and panic attacks. Lavender is analgesic, anti-depressant, antiseptic, anti-viral, decongestant, deodorant, emmenagogic and sedative.

• **Chamomile** This refers to Roman chamomile (Anthemis nobilis), not German chamomile. It is the best essential oil to calm the Throat Chakra, but do not use it if you need to drive a car afterwards, for it can make you feel very 'spaced out'. For most uses, mix 2 drops of the essential oil with 5 ml of base oil. In a vaporizer, chamomile is excellent to ease headaches caused by overwork or stress. It is analgesic, antiseptic, anti-spasmodic, carminative, digestive, diuretic, emmenagogic and sedative.

• **Rosemary/thyme/sage** These three herbs, alone or in combination, make good steam inhalations. However, you should note that they are not recommended for use in home aromatherapy blends, and should not be used at all if you are pregnant.

MAKING A STEAM INHALATION

This type of inhalation makes an excellent treatment for nasal blockages, sinus infections, coughs, colds and sore throats, all of which demonstrate that the Throat Chakra is struggling to keep these minor infections at bay.

1 Boil 1 litre (1¾ pt) of water and pour it into a bowl.

2 Add 10 drops of essential oil (or the fresh herb steeped in water).

3 Put a towel over your head, close your eyes and inhale the vapour for a few minutes at a time, for up to 10 minutes.

Fresh herbs such as lavender, chamomile and rosemary make excellent hot tea infusions or inhalations.

YOGA FOR THE THROAT CHAKRA

Start your yoga session by balancing the chakras with a standing balanced asana (posture) such as Pranamasana (prayer pose). This is simply standing straight with the spine 'lifted', as if a cord is pulling it up from the crown of your head, and placing your hands together in the prayer position.

ACTIVE: BOW

The Bow pose benefits the abdominal area, since in the completed full posture only the abdomen bears the weight of the body. It is also good for the back, bladder and prostate gland. Your breathing will be fast, and from an energetic-flow viewpoint this posture benefits the Throat Chakra. It is common for rising pranic energy to become blocked at the throat, and this asana opens Vishuddha, moving energy up from the abdominal region, thus allowing the release of toxins on all levels. The state of consciousness you are seeking is an objective mental state known as anandamayakosha (the Body of Bliss). Visualize your incoming and outgoing breath as a beautiful turquoise blue light. Picture 1 shows a beginner's asana.

1 Lie on your front, with your face down. Reach back, bending your knees and holding your ankles. Aim to keep your knees together throughout the asana.

2 Pulling on your ankles, slowly and cautiously raise your trunk and legs as high as possible. Stretch your neck. Hold the position.

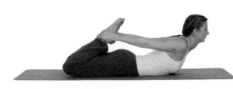

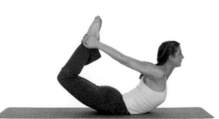

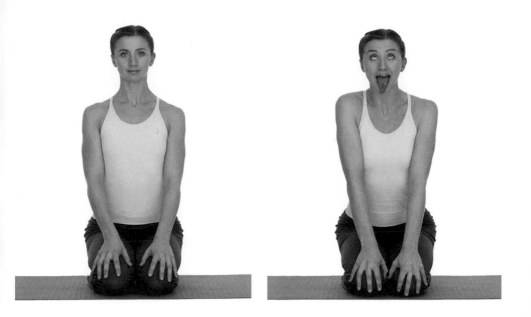

ACTIVE: LION

Despite its strange appearance, this pose needs to be performed with enthusiasm, but without straining. It helps you to learn the three bandhas that control the flow of prana in the physical body, and your speech becomes clearer, too.

This asana is dedicated to Narasimha, the lion-man incarnation of Vishnu (Nara meaning man, and simha meaning lion). Narasimha was a fierce creature who, when called upon, burst out of a pillar in the palace of the evil demon king Hiranya Kasipu, and rescued his pious son Prahlado who was a strong devotee of Vishnu.

1 Either kneel normally or kneel with your knees crossed over (similar to the Cow pose, see page 90). Stretch your trunk forwards, keep your chest open and your back erect. Place your right palm on the right knee and your left palm on the left knee, then straighten your arms and make your fingers into extended 'claws'.

2 Open your jaw wide and stretch your tongue as far as possible towards your chin. Roll your eyes up and gaze towards the centre of your eyebrows. Stay in this posture for about 30 seconds, breathing through your mouth. Repeat with your knees crossed on the opposite side, if applicable.

PASSIVE: SITTING FORWARD BEND

The physical benefits of this pose are similar to those of the Head-to-Knee Forward Bend (see page 109): stretching the backs of the leg muscles and loosening the hip joints, toning the abdominal organs and stretching the spine throughout its entire length. Energy-wise, this asana encourages the upward and downward flow of prana throughout the chakra system towards the Throat Chakra. Visualize the appropriate yantra as you perform it.

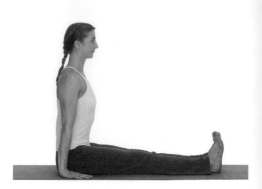

1 Sit on the floor with your legs stretched straight. Place your palms on the floor by the side of your hips. Exhaling, stretch over your legs, bending from the pelvic region. Hold either your ankles or your big toes (whichever you can reach comfortably).

2 Aim to get the back flat but do not overdo the stretch. When you are a beginner at yoga, it is far better to stretch in the general direction of any asana than force the position.

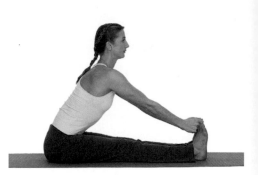

3 With practice you may be able to stretch right over your legs and touch your knees with your nose!

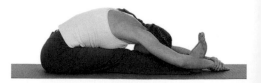

CRYSTALS TO ACTIVATE THE THROAT CHAKRA

Recommended gemstone crystals for activating the Throat Chakra are blue and yellow topaz, each of which are used in slightly different ways.

BLUE TOPAZ

This is an excellent crystal to use when you are ready to activate Vishuddha for deeper spiritual work, or for activation before sacred singing or performing with the voice. Its main purpose is to direct energy, thus aligning the body's meridians. For this reason you can use it sensitively when 'channelling' beneficial entities or Nature spirits, or when you are passing Reiki energy through the body during initiations. It can either be held or worn as jewellery close to the neck.

YELLOW TOPAZ

Use this crystal to activate Vishuddha at a physical level. The energy imbalance that causes hypothyroidism can be 'kick-started' into balance by yellow topaz. It is said to strengthen our nervous system and, through working intensely with Vishuddha, will aid metabolism.

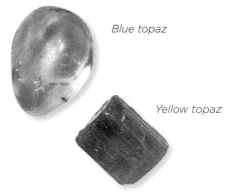

Blue topaz

Yellow topaz

Using topaz to activate vishuddha

You can use either blue or yellow topaz for this exercise. You will need three small uncut topazes and two quartz crystal 'points', 2.5–5 cm (1–2 in) in length.

1 Cleanse the crystals (see page 36) and prepare your healing space by burning some incense or joss-sticks. You can use a special feather fan if you wish to move the smoke into all corners of the room, then let the smoke drift out of an open window.

When you cleanse a room in this way, the smoke bonds with the positive ions in the air that are harmful to us, leaving behind beneficial negative ions. Native Americans developed this cleansing – sometimes called 'smudging' – using sage, cedarwood or sweet scented grass. Those with psychic vision can see that a person's aura is cleared when using fragrant smoke. For auric clearing it is recommended that you start at the head and sweep unwanted energies down the body with the smoke, enabling them to be 'grounded' into Mother Earth.

2 Now lie down on the floor and hold the quartz crystals, one in the centre of each palm, with the points pointing up your arm.

3 Place the three topazes as follows: one in the central notch on your collar bone and one on either side of your neck, pointing inwards.

4 Relax like this for 30 minutes and enjoy your healing session with these crystals.

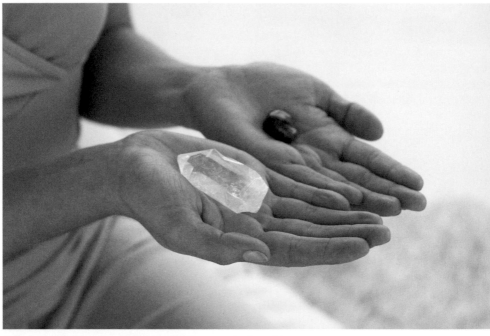

You can activate Vishuddha in a lying or seated position.

CRYSTALS TO CALM THE THROAT CHAKRA

Sapphire (see page 95), emerald (see page 57) and quartz are excellent gemstones to calm the Throat Chakra. All semi-precious gemstones give a high-quality healing vibration that is concentrated and more powerful than that of less precious stones. This is the reason why crystal healers choose to use them rather than the more common tumble-polished stones.

QUARTZ

Light constantly passes through quartz crystals, and bends at 90 degrees as it exits a crystal. This allows full-spectrum light to be transmitted to the body area on which it is placed, enabling the body to draw from it the specific frequencies and harmonics that it requires. For this reason many crystal healers use only clear quartz.

Quartz also displays rainbows of coloured light within it if its structure allows the rays of light to be diffracted by imperfections.

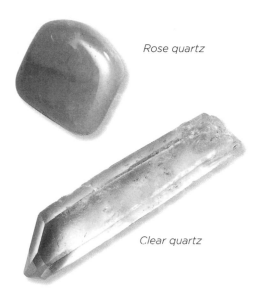

Rose quartz

Clear quartz

Making a gem elixir to calm the throat chakra

An excellent way to calm Vishuddha is to make a gem elixir from sapphire or emerald. You can do this by placing the cleansed crystal in a clear glass of pure spring water and leaving it, covered with a sheet of white paper, in sunshine for three hours. The water is then ready for sipping (remove the crystal first). To potentize it still further, place a number of quartz points around the container, pointing inwards. If you are unable to obtain sapphire or emerald, rose quartz will bring loving energies and calmness into any chakra.

CRYSTALS TO BALANCE THE THROAT CHAKRA

For thousands of years Native American peoples, particularly those of the south-west states where the Hopi people live, have revered crystals. They have a particular affinity with turquoise and instinctively fashioned this soft, easily carved stone into amazing jewellery. They found that when they combined it with silver, lunar energies were increased; when they used it with gold, solar energies were conducted and directed.

TURQUOISE

Turquoise is regarded as the 'stone of the sky'; it is not really a crystal, but is more amorphous in nature. It offers the wearer protection from radiation, particularly when worn around the throat. Amazingly, many Native Americans instinctively knew that the effects of high background radiation from uranium deposits under their lands would be neutralized in their bodies by wearing turquoise stones against the skin.

The amazing clarity of intention with which turquoise stones have evolved helps us to visualize the colour turquoise, which we should see as a clear light bathing us from above being drawn into our Throat Chakra, both at the front and back of the neck. The technique for doing this is called colour breathing.

GEM SILICA AND CHRYSOCOLLA

Today gem silica and chrysocolla are taking the place of turquoise. You can use chrysocolla for dispelling fears, and gem silica makes an excellent calming and balancing stone for Vishuddha. All three stones are very soft and must not be used for making gem elixirs – far better to enjoy them as jewellery, or as healing stones in their own right.

COLOUR BREATHING

This technique is really very simple. You only have to visualize an appropriate colour for each chakra – in this case turquoise for the throat – and feel that you can saturate your breath with that colour. Imagine it being drawn in through your nostrils, passing down your neck and throat into your lungs and chest. When you release your breath, imagine the colour taking away with it any unwanted stagnant energies that cause 'dis-ease'.

The colour blue, when given as light therapy, has been proven to be antiseptic and analgesic in nature. It reduces inflammation and helps congeal the blood. The blue/green colour of turquoise, when given as light therapy, is most appropriate to calm throat and heart conditions.

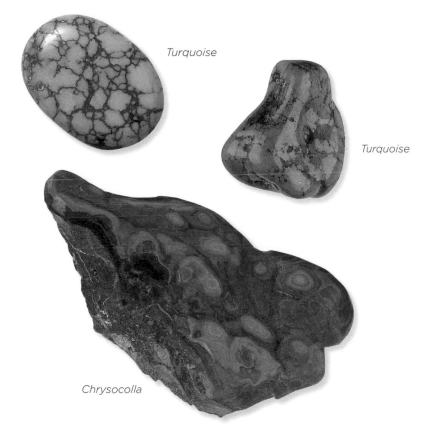

Turquoise

Turquoise

Chrysocolla

THROAT CHAKRA MEDITATION

A good time for meditation is either following yoga practise or after crystal therapy. At such times, your body is already relaxed and ready for a session of focused concentration (see pages 22–23).

BEFORE YOU START

Choose a leisurely and relaxed time to meditate. If you like, create an atmosphere with oils, candles, or incense in the colour of the chakra. Sit or lie somewhere you won't be disturbed. You can pre-record the words of the meditation – dots indicate a pause.

1 Take up a comfortable position and breathe slowly and deeply through your nose.

2 Tense each set of muscles in turn, from feet to your head ... feel yourself sink heavily into the floor or chair ...

3 Now focus on your lower head and neck and imagine a beautiful blue mist washing inside your mouth ... bathing your throat cavity ... swirling around your ears ... caressing your neck ... gliding over your tongue ... relaxing your jaw ... so that the area becomes supple and free ...

AFFIRMATIONS

- I am starting to speak up for myself.

- What I have to say is worthy of being listened to.

- I delight in my self-expression and in all my creative pursuits.

- I listen to and acknowledge the needs and wants of others.

- I always speak from the Heart.

- My thoughts and speech are considered before I utter them.

- My voice is becoming stronger and more compelling.

4 Be aware of tension and draw the attention of this blue mist to that area so it can be released by it ...

5 Be aware of your breathing and allow each inhalation to increase the intensity of the blue mist ... each exhalation to spread this blue mist throughout your throat, mouth, tongue, ears and neck ... strengthening each area ... allowing you to speak your truth ... to express your feelings honestly, openly, with compassion to yourself and others ...

6 As you continue to sense the blue mist swirling around your Throat Chakra think of the words 'I want' and 'I need' ... What do you want?... What do you need? ... You have the right to ask for what you want and what you need ... you have the right to have your demands listened to with respect and patience ...

7 Determine to speak out for yourself in some way every day ...

8 Know that by meditating on this beautiful mist daily you will strengthen and support your Throat Chakra and move toward a time when your needs are listened to ... and met ... Because you have within you everything you need to meet those needs for yourself.

DAILY QUESTIONS

- How could you strengthen your voice? Try singing or reciting a poem in the bath, or chanting each morning for five minutes.

- Does your posture constrict your voice? Try the Alexander Technique to shift negative patterns.

- How could you express your feelings? Start a journal to communicate emotions safely.

- How do you feel about expressing anger? Write to someone you are angry with, but detach yourself from emotion. Imagine your mind full of anger but your Heart as the 'you', offering compassion and love.

- How purified is your body? Take a weekend to cut out stimulants and eat only fresh, raw, steamed, or lightly cooked, food.

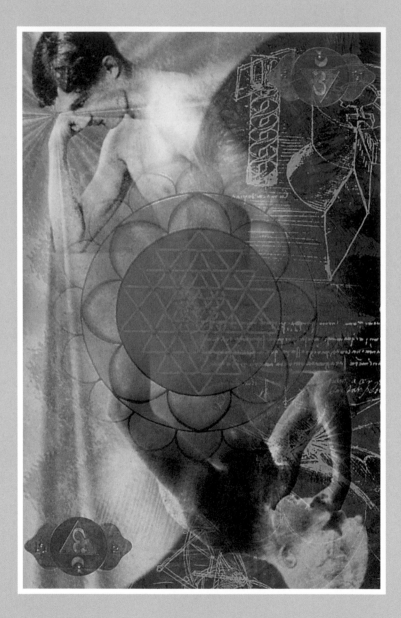

6 THE BROW CHAKRA: AJNA

The Brow Chakra or Ajna is also known as the Third Eye Chakra, the Eye of Shiva, ajita-patra, ajna-pura, jnana-padma, dwidala, bhru chakra and bhruyugamadhyabila. It is linked externally to the physical body just between (and slightly above) the level of the eyebrows.

The word Ajna means 'servant' or 'command' – in the sense of the Guru's command of spiritual guidance. It is referred to as the 'ocean of nectar', the life-sustaining liquid that arises in the mouth of a yogi when he reaches a state of enlightenment. Ajna is depicted with two petals, representing the two aspects of prana that meet here. Its element is Ether.

THE FUNCTIONS OF AJNA

In Tantric yoga, the Brow Chakra is associated with 'manas' or mind, which is beyond even the most subtle elements, although still part of our existence in an Earthly body. In recent Western occult and New Age thought, Ajna has been identified with the 'Third Eye' – our eye of psychic vision, a concept not found in the original Tantric system. When we fully associate ourselves with the power contained within Ajna we are able to step beyond the mind, with all its desires and longings, and enter the realms of knowledge and wisdom. However, if this chakra is blocked, we will confuse information with knowledge; or get carried away with our own powers of insight and use them for our own means or spiritual arrogance.

ADDITIONAL CHAKRAS ASSOCIATED WITH AJNA

Ajna is often described as having at least four distinct minor chakras in a vertical line above it: the Manas, Indu, Mahanada and Nirvana chakras, the last-named being at the top of the head. All combine their energies and resonate with one another to form the Ajna, 'Third Eye' or Eye of Shiva. Another minor chakra, the Soma, contains a triangulation of energy coming from the three main nadis (sushumna, ida and pingala), which combine to make the trinity of Brahma the creator, Vishnu the preserver and Shiva the destroyer.

BROW CHAKRA CORRESPONDENCES

This chart for the Third Eye (Sixth) Chakra identifies all the associations and symbolisms linked with this particular chakra. As such it provides a 'ready reference' of inspirations to use when you carry out practical exercises such as choosing appropriate stones for crystal work.

USING THE CHART

This chart will also help you with the various images that you will need when composing your own meditations and visualizations. Incorporate as many of these symbols and themes as you feel is appropriate to your personal needs.

By reacquainting yourself regularly with this chakra chart as a prelude to the section on the Brow Chakra, you will help to keep your mind focused on related issues, including the awareness of the benefits to be gained from transcending the purely physical world and opening yourself up to intuitive sight and wisdom.

It allows you to tap in to the limitless knowledge which you can access directly in order to answer the questions for which you tend to look to others – be they mentors, gurus, therapists, astrologers, or psychics – to satisfy.

CHAKRA CHARACTERISTICS

See which of the following characteristics of excessive ('too open'), deficient ('blocked'), and balanced chakra energy you can relate to - and then determine (should you choose) to take the necessary action, using the tools and techniques outlined in the following pages of this chapter.

- **Too open** (chakra spins too fast): highly logical, dogmatic, authoritarian, arrogant.

- **Blocked** (chakra spins sluggishly or not at all): undisciplined, fears success, tendency toward schizophrenia, sets sights too low.

- **Balanced** (chakra maintains equilibrium and spins at correct vibrational speed): charismatic, highly intuitive, not attached to material things, may experience unusual phenomena.

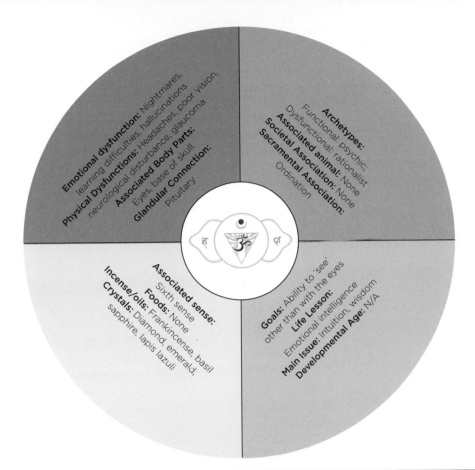

Emotional dysfunction: Nightmares, learning difficulties, hallucinations
Physical Dysfunctions: Headaches, poor vision, neurological disturbance, glaucoma
Associated Body Parts: Eyes, base of skull
Glandular Connection: Pituitary

Archetypes:
Functional: psychic;
Dysfunctional: rationalist
Associated animal: None
Societal Association: None
Sacramental Association: Ordination

Associated sense: Sixth sense
Foods: None
Incense/oils: Frankincense, basil
Crystals: Diamond, emerald, sapphire, lapis lazuli

Goals: Ability to 'see' other than with the eyes
Life Lesson: Emotional intelligence
Main Issue: Intuition, wisdom
Developmental Age: N/A

BROW CHAKRA	
Sanskrit name	Ajna
Meaning	To perceive, to know
Location	Above and between eyebrows
Symbol	Lotus with two large petals on either side, resembling eyes or wings (see page 140 for the yantra)
Associated colours	Indigo
Element	Light/telepathic energy
Ruling planet	Jupiter

BROW CHAKRA YANTRA

*Ajna is like the moon, beautifully white. It shines with the glory of meditation.
Within this lotus dwells the subtle mind. When the yogi ... becomes
dissolved in this place, which is the abode of uninterrupted bliss,
he then sees sparks of fire distinctly shining.*

— Sat Cakra Nirupana

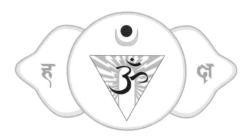

DESCRIPTION OF THE YANTRA

- **Number of petals:** The Ajna mantra is depicted as having two large petals. They represent the duality that is present in all things.

- **Colour:** White or deep blue.

- **Mantras:** Within each petal is a mantra. 'Hang', representing Shiva, is on one side. 'Ksham', representing Shakti, is on the other side. Together they form the phrase 'I am that I am'.

- **White circle:** At the centre of the yantra, a white circle represents the void.

- **Downward-pointing triangle:** Within the white circle, there is a downward-pointing triangle, which contains the mantra OM and a lingam (phallus).

- **Quarter moon:** A quarter moon shown at the top of the yantra, this indicates a vortex of energy.

- **Bindu:** The dot symbolizes complete detachment from our female or male body. Showing control of the body, it has managed to rise above the triangle that represents sexual energy in an 'impure' state.

BROW CHAKRA ARCHETYPES

The following story illustrates perfectly the functional and dysfunctional archetypes of the Brow Chakra. Say the opportunity comes up to write a book on an unfamiliar subject, yet the author knows immediately that they are destined to do it. The two sides of the brain wrestle for supremacy before the author can take action.

The left, logical, hemisphere 'suggests' that the subject is perhaps not quite right. But the right, creative, side simply trusts that writing the book is the way forward. The author opts to write the book, which is a huge success and eventually leads the author into a period of growth.

THE RATIONALIST

Had the author allowed his/her intellect to override his/her intuition he/she would never have directed his/her career on to a path that is offered both material and spiritual satisfaction and success. Yet how common it is for us to give way to the Rationalist inside all of us? This dysfunctional archetype allows the left brain dominance, usually because of the fear and insecurity we feel at dismantling the safe world in which we have become cocooned and constricted. In reality, Rationalists are not simply people who take a 'scientific' view of everything. This group also embraces controllers and perfectionists – those who cannot accept the human failings of others and are similarly hard on themselves.

THE PSYCHIC

The functional archetype of this chakra is the Psychic, which doesn't just refer to those people who use their powers in a professional sense, but anyone who trusts that the answers to life's challenges lie within themselves. Having been awakened to the need to listen by developing the Throat (Fifth) Chakra, Psychics now listen to their inner Self. They recognize that the wisdom of the Brow Chakra is like a whisper that cannot be heard unless the cacophony of everyday life is stilled. Hence they recognize the need for meditation and contemplation in order for their creativity and intuition to shine through.

BROW CHAKRA AROMATHERAPY

Passion flower, papaya and tarragon are recommended for Ajna. Passion flower, either as a herbal preparation or as a flower essence, is used to alleviate neuralgia and insomnia. As a fruit, papaya settles digestive-system disturbances, while its flower essence reminds people of their karmic lessons. Tarragon, as a fresh herb, is diuretic and digestive as a hot tea infusion with a little honey; as a flower essence it stimulates this chakra and assists self-expression and insight.

BROW CHAKRA ESSENTIAL OILS

The main essential oils that have a sympathetic resonance with Ajna are:

- **Frankincense** Also called olibanum, Frankincense has a wonderful spicy perfume extracted from the resinous gum of a small North African tree. It has been used for centuries as an embalming oil.

  Today its golden, gummy pieces still form the main ingredient of the incense burned in Christian churches. You can burn frankincense directly on special charcoal discs, or use the thick amber-coloured essential oil in a vaporizer. Its properties assist deep meditation and focus on the Brow Chakra. Frankincense promotes a feeling of profound relaxation and deepens awareness of the breath, taking you into dream states where past memories may more easily be accessed. For the physical body, as well as benefiting respiratory infections and asthma, Frankincense helps to slow down and deepen the breathing and is best used as gentle chest massage, which also helps to open the often-constricted chest area. Frankincense also promotes new skin and cells, is anti-inflammatory, antiseptic, astringent, carminative, digestive, diuretic, expectorant and sedative.

- **Basil and holy basil** An aromatic herb much used in Italian cooking, basil was once powdered and taken as snuff. As an essential oil, it is excellent in a vaporizer to clear the head and give strength, helping to balance Ajna, Vishuddha and the minor head chakras. Basil was valued in medieval times as part of a blend for anointing the heads of

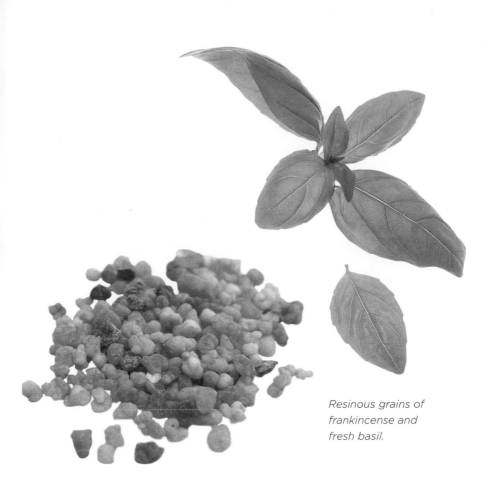

Resinous grains of frankincense and fresh basil.

kings and queens during coronation ceremonies and was called the 'royal herb'.

Basil is effective for nervous disorders, poor memory, lack of concentration and headaches caused by congestion. Basil tea is recommended to sober you up if you are drunk! As massage oil, it is best as a blend with lemon and geranium and should never be used excessively; it should not be used as bath oil as it may cause skin irritation; avoid any use of basil throughout pregnancy. Basil is antiseptic, anti-spasmodic, carminative, digestive, emmenagogic, febrifuge and a nerve tonic.

YOGA FOR THE BROW CHAKRA

Start your yoga session by balancing the chakras with a standing balanced asana (posture) such as Pranamasana (prayer pose). This is simply standing straight with the spine 'lifted', as if a cord is pulling it up from the crown of your head, and placing your hands together in the prayer position.

ACTIVE:
DOG FACE-DOWN POSE

This asana is particularly useful to gently prepare you for headstands, because you get used to the extra blood flow to the head. Energy-wise, you should concentrate on the Third Eye while you hold the pose for as long as possible. Alternatively, visualize a deep-blue light.

1 Kneel on all fours, then 'walk' your hands further forwards, with your palms flat on the floor.

2 Raise your trunk, straightening your legs and keeping your feet flat on the floor. Pull in your abdomen. Your head should relax down in line with your arms and body. The shape of this asana is an inverted V.

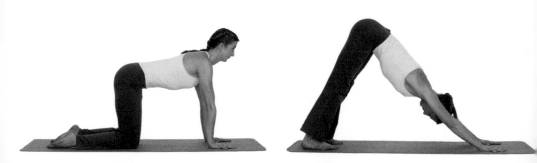

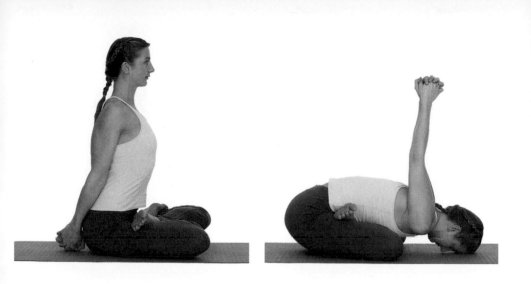

ACTIVE: YOGA MUDRA IN PADMASANA

This advanced pose is traditionally performed in Padmasana (the lotus position), but if this is difficult you can use a simple crossed-leg position. You need to suspend your breathing while you are in the mudra (work towards one minute) and maintain your focus on Ajna, the Brow Chakra.

Only perform this once in each yoga programme. The purpose of this mudra is to cleanse the nadis to support the esoteric practices of Hatha yoga. By focusing on Ajna you render the entire energy field ready for concentration/meditation (dharana/dhyana). The state of consciousness you are seeking is the intuitive state, for your Soul Body is nourished by intuition.

1 Sit with your legs crossed in the full lotus posture. Clasp your hands behind your back, locking your fingers together.

2 On an exhalation, bend forward and touch the top of your head to the floor (or as near as possible). Simultaneously raise your arms straight up behind your back. Hold for as long as possible without breathing.

PASSIVE: PLOUGH POSE

The physical benefits of this asana are numerous: the bowels move freely, the spine becomes flexible, all the internal organs benefit, and increased blood flow at the neck improves thyroid and parathyroid hormone production.

From an energy-flow viewpoint, this asana is supreme, toning all the chakras at the same time. Once mastered, this is also one of the most relaxing asanas. It gives you plenty of time to focus on moving energy into your Brow Chakra. If this pose is new to you, you can support your back with your hands or rest your legs on a chair/stool positioned at the correct height and distance behind your head (the assistance of a friend or teacher is helpful). It is important to follow this asana with a backward bend, such as the fish pose, see page 110).

1 Lie flat on your back, with your legs stretched out and tight at the knees. Supporting your back, bend your knees, raise your hips from the floor and lift your trunk up perpendicularly, supported by your hands, until your chest touches your chin. Move your hands to the middle of your spine. Your legs should be straight with your toes pointing up.

2 Release the chin lock and lower your trunk slightly. Stretch your arms out on the floor and simultaneously move your legs up over your head, resting your toes on the floor behind it. Your legs should be together throughout and straight. Remain in this asana from one to five minutes, breathing normally. To come out of the pose, support your back and lower your knees as you bring them over your head to the floor.

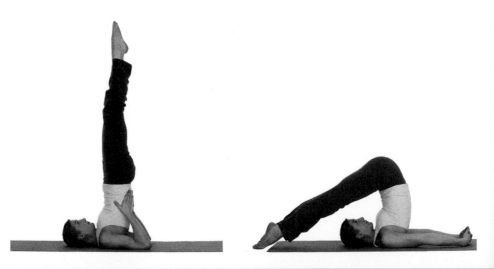

CRYSTALS TO ACTIVATE
THE BROW CHAKRA

Perhaps you would like to develop your intuitional powers, your insight, imagination and clairvoyance? Then Ajna is the chakra to work with – provided the lower chakras are already in balance. It really is not beneficial to have a highly developed Third Eye if you have not yet come to grips with the basic life functions that manifest through the Base Chakra, for example.

DIAMONDS

These beautiful precious gemstones need no introduction. However, they assist us to move into deeper levels. They are one of the finest examples of the crystal world gifted to us from Mother Nature, displaying all her beauty and timelessness.

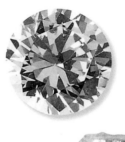

Faceted diamond

If we wear diamonds as jewellery, their power enlarges and strengthens our energy field – whether we are a calm, happy person or a sad one. Whatever our emotions, they will be amplified in the astral/emotional levels of the aura; and whatever our mental processes, they will be amplified in the mental level. When we choose to wear diamonds for meditation, we amplify our aura in the areas where potent spiritual essences lie, around our spiritual and causal bodies.

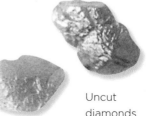

Uncut diamonds

HERKIMER DIAMOND

If you are unable to use authentic diamonds for your healing work, then a lovely, naturally faceted crystal (a type of quartz) is Herkimer diamond. 'Herkies', as they are known, are clear and very hard – almost as hard as diamonds – and they are nearly always double-terminated (with points at both ends).

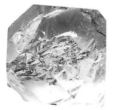

Herkimer protects from geopathic stress, balances energetic cellular disorders and helps to access past-life memories.

Using a herkie for activation

Only attempt to activate the Brow Chakra on yourself – do not do this to others unless you are a trained healer.

1 Rub your Third Eye area briskly.

2 Lie down, placing a Herkie on the Third Eye and relax. If you are ready for it, the crystal may assist in bringing you visions or guidance.

For any deep spiritual work, it is always best to have a clear intention of what you are seeking, and to form that intention in your mind. When that intention is clear, bright and shining (just like a diamond), you may be rewarded with extraordinary levels of perception. This activation can be made more powerful by resting Herkies on either side of your head, level with your temples. The temples are minor chakras - indeed, they function as temples in our head, standing one on each side of the skull ready to receive offerings, with Vishuddha calling from below and Sahasrara, the Crown Chakra, beckoning from above.

CRYSTALS TO CALM THE BROW CHAKRA

We need to look at why you might want to calm Ajna. Perhaps you have constant headaches brought on by a stressful lifestyle; or cannot come to terms with new ideas that throw your comfortable views of life into disarray.

Calming does not necessarily mean suppressing anything of a spiritual nature, but makes for a harmonious flow of radiance into whatever you choose to do that is of a higher nature. Sapphire and emerald are the calming stones for Ajna.

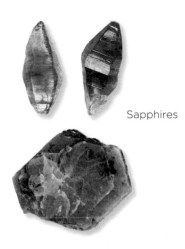
Sapphires

EMERALD

Emerald calms Ajna because of its colour vibration. When you go to sleep, tape a small piece of emerald to your Third Eye to help settle issues that have been brought just below the surface in uncomfortable dreams. Use emerald for headaches too, making it into a gem elixir or holding the crystal during meditation.

SAPPHIRE

Using sapphire in the same way as emerald, by taping it to the Third Eye, brings deep insight into matters of a spiritual nature. Insights can then be processed by your whole body–mind–spirit complex, for in this incarnation you have been given the gift of having a physical body and a mind that responds to fantasy, suggestion and symbols.

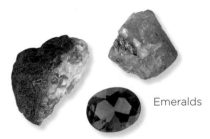
Emeralds

CRYSTALS TO BALANCE
THE BROW CHAKRA

Historically, Ajna has had a very special 'love affair' with lapis lazuli. This crystal was used in a number of ancient cultures (including Atlantis) to balance a person's highest spiritual powers.

If we could part the mists of time and peer into the distant past, we would find that people were once much more spiritually developed then than they are today. They had bodies of a finer etheric substance, and it is said that in the times when beautiful temples were built, the gods and goddesses could enter into them in spirit and manifest visible bodies of Light. Everywhere people could communicate easily with animals, trees, flowers and crystals. As Rudolph Steiner (the 20th-century founder of anthroposophy) put it, 'The intention of the Graeco-Roman race was to charm Spirit into Matter.'

Today, however, the tables seem to be turned and we have dense etheric bodies, but the reality is that we have to experience this densification before we can return our energy bodies to the Light.

LAPIS LAZULI

Good-quality lapis lazuli is a deep blue stone, with little gold flecks of iron pyrites sparkling within it like stars. It is sometimes called the 'night stone' for this reason. It is found mainly in India and Afghanistan, both areas of rich cultural and spiritual heritage. It was used extensively in the tomb of Tutankhamun for decoration, and by ancient Egyptian women to make blue eye shadow.

The effects of lapis lazuli

Working strongly and energetically, lapis lazuli strengthens both the thyroid and parathyroid glands, and our skeletal system, in which the history of the body is locked. It is also said to benefit energy depletions that cause hearing loss, blood and nervous disorders.

On a mental/emotional level, lapis lazuli is used at Ajna to access our deep cellular memory, our hurts and fears, and to bring them into acceptance in our lives through the wisdom of higher consciousness. Whenever this occurs, we are better able to cope with whatever life deals out to us.

One way to experience the stunning energies of lapis lazuli is to make a crystal essence using the indirect method (see page 39). It is too soft a stone to put into water using the direct method, because it contains an unstable mixture of minerals.

How to use lapis lazuli

Lapis lazuli is a powerful healer and balancer for the energies of Ajna and it will benefit you to spend time getting to know its qualities.

1 Cleanse the lapis carefully, but not with water (as it is a 'soft' stone), instead with your intention by holding it in the palm of you hand and breathing gently upon it. In this way the pranic energy in your breath does the cleansing.

2 Now hold the stone to your Third Eye and 'ask' to understand the lapis. It may be that colours or pictures will come into your head or you may receive a message directly from the crystal. Whatever it is, thank the lapis before disconnecting your energy from it.

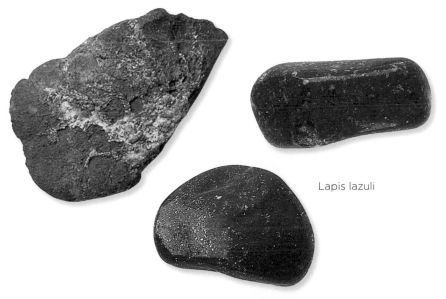

Lapis lazuli

BROW CHAKRA MEDITATION

A good time for meditation is either following yoga practise or after crystal therapy. At such times, your body is already relaxed and ready for a session of focused concentration (see pages 22–23).

BEFORE YOU START

Choose a leisurely and relaxed time to meditate. If you like, create an atmosphere with oils, candles, or incense in the colour of the chakra. Sit or lie somewhere you won't be disturbed. You can pre-record the words of the meditation – dots indicate a pause.

1 Assume a comfortable position and breathe slowly and deeply through your nose.

2 Tense each set of muscles in turn, from the feet and ankles to the neck and head ... and as they relax feel yourself sink heavily into the floor or the chair ...

3 In your mind's eye become aware of the Third Eye Chakra, positioned between your eyebrows, as if it were a physical entity ...

4 Focus on the twin white wings of the Ajna symbol on either side of a circle (see page 140) ...

AFFIRMATIONS

- I recognize the need for silence and stillness in my life.

- The answers to all my questions lie within me.

- I trust my inner self to guide and protect me.

- I trust my feelings.

- I have nothing to prove.

- I am full of wisdom.

- I trust that my imagination will create a world of happiness and security for me.

- Imagination is the life-blood of my creativity.

- I choose to accept myself and others exactly as we are.

See the golden triangle within that circle, pointing downward toward the earth ... connecting your Higher Consciousness with your physical entity ...

5 Now flood that symbol with the colour indigo so that it bathes your forehead with violet-blue ... violet washing down from the Crown Chakra at the top of your head ... and blue moving up from the Throat Chakra at the base of your neck ...

6 Your Third Eye Chakra is a beautiful lotus flower ... feel its roots go deep within your forehead, connecting with the Sushumna, the central column linking the stems of each chakra ...

7 Feel the energy of the Third Eye vortex as it spins effortlessly between your physical eyes ... sense the pulsation of chakra energy ...

8 Be very aware of any other sensations you may experience – smell the fragrance of the Third Eye Chakra lotus ...

9 The Third Eye is as real as your two physical eyes ... it is there to offer you insight, clairvoyance, truths to the questions of the universe ... nurture it as carefully as you would your physical eyes ... exercise it daily ... let your intuition guide you daily, leading you to a more fulfilling, joyous life. Stay relaxed as you return to your normal surroundings.

DAILY QUESTIONS

- How much silence is there in your life for the whispers of intuition to be heard? Spend time in silence. Focus on something beautiful and be still and silent.

- When did you last act on intuition? Go with any compelling thoughts, without rationalization. Be alert to coincidences and experiences that may contain messages.

- Do you truly see what is around you? Exercise your physical perception by being alert to details, such as shapes and colours.

- Do you look outside yourself for answers? List personal queries, such as why a certain person has come into your life. Note insights in the form of images, colours, words, or phrases.

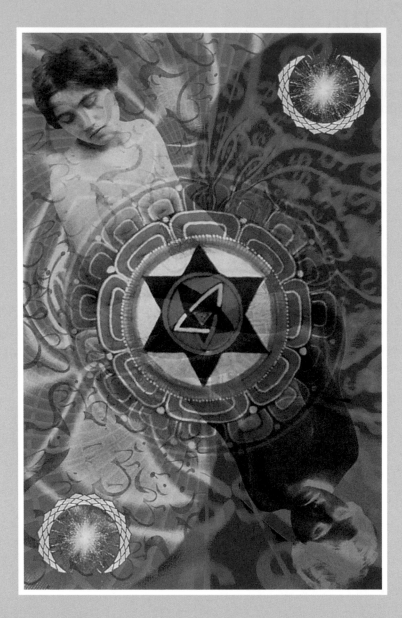

7 THE CROWN CHAKRA: SAHASRARA

The Crown Chakra or Sahasrara is also known as the Thousand-petalled Lotus, akasha chakra, sahasrara padma, sahasrara mahapadma, sahasrara saroruha, sahasradala, sahasradala padma, pankaja, kamala, adhomukha mahapadma, wyomambhoja, shiras padma, amlana padma, dashashatadala padma, shuddha padma and shantyatita pada.

Sahasrara, which means 'a thousand petals', is described in Indian traditions as being placed above the head, while more modern theosophical thinking locates it at the top of the head. Mystics describe its 1,000 white petals being arranged in 20 layers, each containing 50 petals with letters of the Sanskrit (an ancient holy language) alphabet written on them. The colours of these petals changes as a shimmering rainbow of colours passes through them, although in the seven-chakra system the Crown Chakra is assigned the colour of violet.

THE FUNCTIONS OF SAHASRARA

Sahasrara is the place of pure consciousness. The Crown Chakra symbolizes the balance of duality within us and our ability to experience super-consciousness, and then the bliss of transcendental consciousness. Because this state is impossible to describe, it is sometimes called 'the Void'. Perhaps the best way to begin to understand it is to enter regularly into deep meditation, where you let go of everything and find that all is peace.

ADDITIONAL CHAKRAS IN THE TANTRIC SYSTEM

- **The Forehead Chakra** – also called Indu or Chandra (Moon) – has 16 petals, is white and 'blossoms' when we achieve exemplary spiritual consciousness.

- **The Tantric Lower Forehead Centre** is also known as the Manas (Mind) Chakra. It has six petals that are normally white, but assume other colours associated with the five senses, plus mind.

These chakras are located between Ajna and Sahasrara.

CROWN CHAKRA CORRESPONDENCES

This chart for the Crown (Seventh) Chakra identifies all the associations and symbolisms linked with this particular chakra. As such it provides a 'ready reference' of inspirations to use when you carry out practical exercises such as choosing appropriate stones for crystal work.

USING THE CHART

This chart will also help you with the various images you will need when composing your own meditations and visualizations. Incorporate as many of these symbols and themes as you feel is appropriate to your needs.

By reacquainting yourself regularly with this chakra chart as a prelude to the section on the Crown Chakra, you will help to keep your mind focused on related issues, including the reprogramming of dysfunctional patterns of thought and behaviour.

Your journey through the chakras has led you to a new horizon and from this spiritual perspective has expanded your consciousnesses, so that you live a more fulfilled, joyous, and healthy life.

CHAKRA CHARACTERISTICS

See which of the following characteristics of excessive ('too open'), deficient ('blocked'), and balanced chakra energy you can relate to – and then determine (should you choose) to take the necessary action, using the tools and techniques outlined in this chapter.

- **Too open** (chakra spins too fast): psychotic or manic depressive, confused sexual expression, frustrated, sense of unrealized power.

- **Blocked** (chakra spins sluggishly or not at all): constantly exhausted, can't make decisions, no sense of 'belonging'.

- **Balanced** (chakra maintains equilibrium and spins at correct vibrational speed): magnetic personality, achieves 'miracles' in life, transcendent, at peace with self.

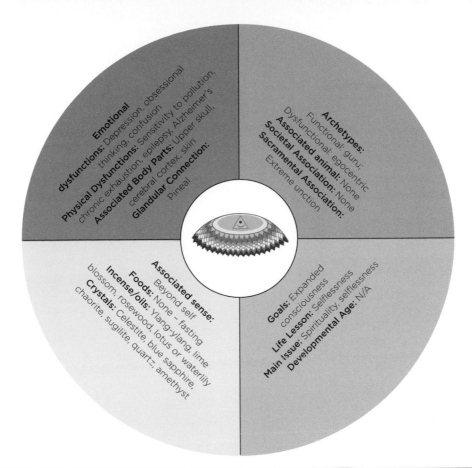

Emotional
dysfunctions: Depression, obsessional
thinking, confusion
Physical Dysfunctions: Sensitivity to pollution,
chronic exhaustion, epilepsy, Alzheimer's
Associated Body Parts: Upper skull,
cerebral cortex, skin
Glandular Connection:
Pineal

Archetypes:
Functional: guru
Dysfunctional: egocentric
Associated animal: None
Societal Association: None
Sacramental Association:
Extreme unction

Associated sense:
Beyond self
Foods: None – fasting
Incense/oils: Ylang-ylang, lime
blossom, rosewood, lotus or waterlily
Crystals: Celestite, blue sapphire,
chaorite, sugilite, quartz, amethyst

Goals: Expanded
consciousness
Life Lesson: Selflessness
Main Issue: Spirituality, selflessness
Developmental Age: N/A

CROWN CHAKRA	
Sanskrit name	Sahasrara
Meaning	Thousandfold
Location	Top/crown of head
Symbol	The 1000-petalled lotus flower (see page 158 for the yantra).
Associated colours	Violet, gold, white
Element	Thought, cosmic energy
Ruling planet	Uranus

CROWN CHAKRA YANTRA

The lotus of the thousand petals, lustrous and whiter than the full moon, has its head turned downward. It charms. It sheds its rays in profusion and is moist and cool like nectar. That most excellent of men who has controlled his mind and known this place is never again born the Wandering, as there is nothing in the three worlds which binds him.

— Sat Cakra Nirupana

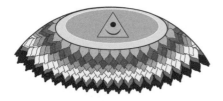

DESCRIPTION OF THE YANTRA

- **Number of petals:** The Sahasrara yantra has one thousand petals.

- **Colour:** Violet

- **Form:** The Sahasrara yantra has a bell-shaped form and can be shown on a yogi's head. The form is associated with Divine knowledge and enlightenment. It is often shown as an open lotus.

- **Mandala**: At the centre of the Sahasrara yantra are two discs or mandala – one inside the other.

The first mandala is Chandra (the Moon) and the second mandala is Surya (the Sun).

- **Triangle:** Within the Chandra mandala is a yellow, upward-pointing triangle.

- **Nirvana-kala:** Inside the yellow triangle sits the Nirvana-kala, said to grant the power of Divine knowledge

- **Supreme bindu:** Above the Nirvana-kala, the supreme bindu stands for the silence led into by the sound of OM

- **The lotus flower:** The lotus flower has been used as a symbol of the chakras because it looks rather like flower blossoms within the auric field. The lotus flower has been a potent emblem in India for thousands of years.

CROWN CHAKRA ARCHETYPES

Success and spirituality are not mutually exclusive. However, when the former is sought at the expense of the latter the resulting imbalanced state illustrates the difference between the positive and negative archetypes of the Crown (Seventh) Chakra – the Guru and the Egocentric

THE EGOCENTRIC

Egocentrics regard themselves as wholly responsible for all the benefits they accrue in life. Indeed, their psychological well-being largely depends on material success, since Egocentrics identify themselves solely in terms of what they do, not who they are. The problem is that they are so busy focusing on their destination that they neglect to enjoy the journey and their tendency to workaholism often leaves them lonely and unfulfilled at the deepest level.

The Egocentric world view is mechanistic in that they have no time for anything that cannot be explained logically. Hence they fail to draw benefit from all that is mysterious and inexplicable in life. It is sometimes only late in life, when the trappings of success – particularly status at work – have been stripped from them through retirement or redundancy (or their health suffers because of their relentless 'good living' lifestyle), that Egocentrics are forced to confront their spiritual bankruptcy.

THE GURU

Gurus take an expansive view of their world situation. They may focus on specific, attainable, goals, but know that there are infinite possibilities – more than the human mind alone can fathom – through which those goals might be realized. Therefore they are open to, and embrace, the unexpected, the serendipitous, the coincidental. Unlike the arrogant, self-centred Egocentric, Gurus accept how little they know and trust that their connection to their Higher Self will always provide the right answer or pathway. These individuals radiate an inner calm that comes from a total acceptance of who – not what – they truly are. These are not human beings trying to be spiritual, but spiritual beings learning vital emotional lessons through temporarily wearing the cloak of humanity.

CROWN CHAKRA AROMATHERAPY

Various plants, herbs and flower essences are used for the Crown Chakra, including yam, witch hazel, comfrey, hawthorn and lavender. Lobelia now used sparingly as a herbal tincture was once smoked in Native American peace-pipe ceremonies. It is a 'nervine' so acts as a tonic to stimulate and strengthen the nervous system.

CROWN CHAKRA ESSENTIAL OILS

The following essential oils are used for their emotional-spiritual properties – not for physical ailments. The first three may be used as aphrodisiac/moisturizing baths: put just two or three drops of each into a carrier oil or milk, then mix it into the warm water.

- **Ylang-ylang** This is a highly perfumed exotic flower that grows mainly in the Far East. In aromatherapy it aids relaxation, calmness and sensuality, although too high a concentration of ylang-ylang will bring on headaches. In cooperation with the unseen flower beings, whom we can petition through prayer, meditation or song, ylang-ylang will open us to Gaia Earth Mother.

- **Rosewood** This is sometimes replaced with other fragrances because the trees that grow in tropical Brazil and Peru have become an endangered species. However, it is possible to buy this essential oil from wood that has been cultivated in sustainable plantations. Rosewood connects and grounds the Root Chakra with the Crown Chakra. Again, seek the cooperation of the unseen worlds when using this essential oil with the Crown Chakra.

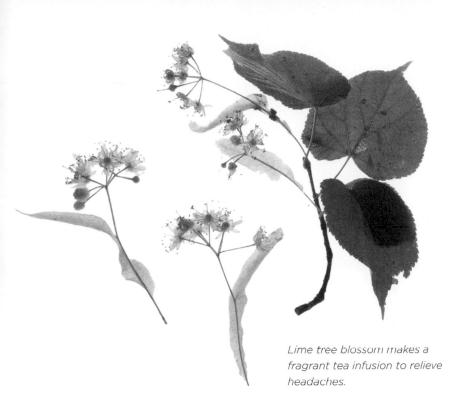

Lime tree blossom makes a fragrant tea infusion to relieve headaches.

• **Linden or lime blossom** This comes not from the citrus fruit, but from the tree *Tilia vulgaris*, and is a highly concentrated perfume ideal for opening the channelling circuit that runs in a 'loop' between the Brow, Alta Major and Throat Chakras. This creates the conditions of relaxation and concentration necessary for removing awareness of our everyday mind processes, in preparation for entering into an altered state of consciousness. When this occurs, some sensitive people are able to 'channel' Beings of Light, including angels and ascended masters and those who guide us from other realms. Linden will also open us up to channel nature spirits and devas/angels of the landscape.

• **Lotus or water lily** This is one of the most rare essential oils. The properties gifted to us by the 'flower beings' of lotus and water lily immediately open the Crown Chakra, bringing an almost hypnotic state of bliss. If you are unable to obtain the essential oil, lotus is sometimes available as an (unperfumed) flower essence.

YOGA FOR THE CROWN CHAKRA

Start your yoga session by balancing the chakras with a standing balanced asana (posture) such as Pranamasana (prayer pose). This is simply standing straight with the spine 'lifted', as if a cord is pulling it up from the crown of your head, and placing your hands together in the prayer position.

You then proceed, undertaking the recommended asanas, and end your yoga session with a balanced sitting asana, such as Sirhasana (simple sitting posture), Siddhasana or Padmasana (lotus posture), or lying down in Savasana (corpse/relaxation pose).

ACTIVE: HEADSTAND

If you have never done a headstand before, always prepare yourself first with asanas such as the Plough pose (see page 146) or the Dog Face-down pose (see page 144) for a number of months until you are completely comfortable with them. Some teachers advise a year of regular yoga practice before attempting a full headstand. Do not do this asana if you have high or low blood pressure; instead begin very gently and slowly with the Plough. Once mastered, the headstand and its variations are regarded as the most beneficial asanas. The headstand is known as the king of all asanas because it makes for healthy blood flow through the brain cells, thus increasing longevity and benefiting the pineal and pituitary glands, which act as a bridge to the higher chakras. So the Crown Chakra is particularly energized by this asana.

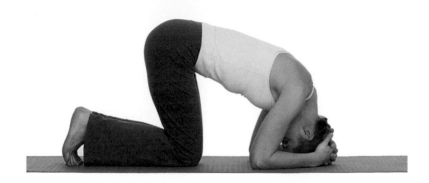

1 Fold up a blanket and place it
in front of you, then kneel on all
fours. Rest your forearms on the
centre of the blanket. Cup your
fingers together and lock them, as
they will be supporting your weight.
Rest the crown of your head on the
blanket, supported by your hands.

2 Raise your knees from the floor
by moving your toes closer to
your head. When you are ready, lift
your trunk and bend your knees.
Straighten your legs and balance.

Caution: This advanced asana is only
for those who can balance safely. If
you have a medical condition, do not
attempt extreme asanas unless you
have taken medical advice and are
working with a qualified yoga teacher.

PASSIVE: SHOULDER STAND

If you move into this pose from the plough, you can maintain the strong chin lock that is the main feature for subtle-energy control; this also facilitates comfort for the physical body. The inversion of the torso is reputed to assist numerous bodily functions. From a subtle-energy viewpoint, it allows the free flow of energies through the body until they reach the neck. At this point prana is able to flow into the brain, while there is a restriction of blood flow into it. When the posture is released, blood again flows freely to the brain.

The Crown Chakra responds to energetic stimulation by an outpouring of sparkling golden white light. You may wish to concentrate on your Crown and visualize this as a fountain of light at the top of your head whenever you are in a Crown Chakra asana.

1 Lie flat on your back, with your legs stretched out and tight at the knees. Supporting your back, bend your knees.

2 Raise your hips from the floor and lift your trunk up perpendicularly, supported by your hands, until your chest touches your chin.

3 Move your hands to the middle of your spine. Your legs should be straight with your toes pointing up. Remain in this position for up to five minutes, breathing evenly. Aim to balance on your shoulders and be still – do not turn your head.

Caution: Only practise this pose under the guidance of a yoga teacher, since there are potential dangers associated with it if you suffer from high blood pressure, and during menstruation. If you have a medical condition, do not attempt extreme asanas without taking medical advice.

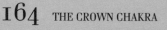

CRYSTALS TO ACTIVATE THE CROWN CHAKRA

There are two principal crystals used to activate the Crown Chakra. They are celestite and blue sapphire.

CELESTITE

Celestite is often called the 'stone of heaven' and is a pale blue translucent crystal that works at a highly refined rate of vibration. It is the most powerfully beautiful expression of blue light known on the Earth. In the physical body it reduces stress by aiding relaxation into the realms of Divine Light. It will also work through additional chakras beyond the traditional seven to alter your physical rate of vibration and result in an 'upgrading' of your web of life. A spiritually aware person will understand this as the true destiny for human beings, although others will subconsciously resist change.

Celestite is excellent made into a crystal essence using the indirect method (see page 39). It can also be held in the hand during meditation or placed on an altar to focus the pure aqua ray of light into the Earth, where its peacefulness is currently much needed.

BLUE SAPPHIRE

Blue sapphire freely gives of its energies to activate all the higher chakras, and delights in its manifestation of an intense, focused blue light.

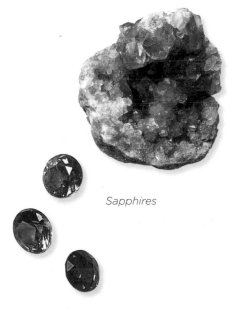

Sapphires

Exercise to experience the energies of blue sapphire

You will need a small blue sapphire (uncut is fine) and a clear quartz point about 5 cm (2 in) long. Ask the deva (the overlighting presence) of each crystal if you may use them to assist your spiritual growth. Find a quiet space. Ensure that you have cleansed and dedicated your crystals first – also always cleanse them after any healing work. Now you can begin.

1 Place a protective circle of light around yourself, by visualizing breathing pure white light into your body through your Crown Chakra, then passing from your hands (held in the prayer position) around your entire body.

2 Place the sapphire in your non-dominant hand, letting it nestle in the centre of the palm, where there is a minor chakra. Hold the quartz in your other palm, ensuring that its point is directed towards your wrist, so that the energy will flow up your arm.

3 Now relax, breathe deeply and start to visualize the condition of your Throat Chakra, then of your Third Eye and finally of your Crown Chakra. Draw the pure blue light of the sapphire into each chakra in turn.

4 When you have finished, offer thanks for the healing gift and ensure that each chakra is balanced and that you have grounded yourself to the Earth.

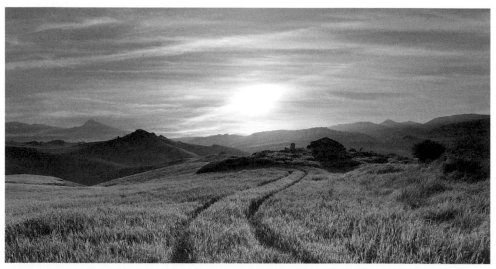

Being outdoors in nature can intensify your experience of the energies.

CRYSTALS TO CALM THE CROWN CHAKRA

Emerald (see page 57) is recommended to calm the energies of Sahasrara, if you wish to switch your focus from spiritual matters to everyday ones.

CHAROITE AND SUGILITE

These types of crystals can be used interchangeably as both have similar qualities to share with humans. It is only in recent years that these stones have been revealed to us by the Earth. They range in colour from pale to deep violet, sometimes with the inclusion of darker minerals.

Although they are not normally classed as gemstones, both charoite and sugilite are regarded as stones of transformation with particular affinities to Sahasrara. The crystalline worlds of these transformational stones are able to convert any negative energies coming into the chakra, in the form of psychic attacks that may manifest as nightmares.

Benefits for the Crown Chakra Charoite crystals encourage deep sleep and assists energetic disturbances of the brain, such as those resulting from autism and deep emotional problems. Sugulite (also known as luvulite) is an excellent crystal to use for learning

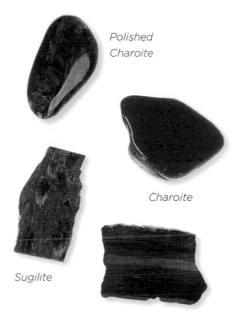

Polished Charoite

Charoite

Sugilite

Luvulite

difficulties as it is said to reorganize brain patterns. In this respect it will clear headaches, purify the blood and lymph, and is considered beneficial in easing the energetic disturbances of epilepsy – all of these disorders have been associated with a malfunctioning and unbalanced Sahasrara or Crown Chakra.

CRYSTALS TO BALANCE THE CROWN CHAKRA

Clear quartz and amethyst, either alone or in combination, are excellent to balance the energies of Sahasrara.

CLEAR QUARTZ

This crystal exists in many forms and shapes. The quartz recommended for using with the chakras is a clear quartz 'point' that measures about 5 cm (2 in) long. It can be single-terminated (with a point at one end) or double-terminated (a point at both ends). It can be shiny and polished or in its natural state.

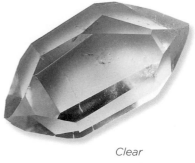

Clear quartz

For some deep shamanic-type healing, the clearer the crystal, the better. If you wish to develop powers beyond the Crown Chakra, then clear quartz is the crystal to assist you.

QUARTZ TO PROTECT YOUR HIGHER CHAKRAS

When working with your higher chakras, it is recommended that you wear a quartz point as a piece of jewellery. It should hang around your neck, resting on your chest, with the point facing down towards the Earth. Place the crystal in the position known to some Native American healers as 'the spiritual grounding point': right at the end of the breastbone between the Heart Chakra and Solar Plexus Chakra. Doing this will always keep your electromagnetic field or aura perfectly clear. Anything negative coming near you will be repelled by light transmitted through the quartz. Always choose your crystal jewellery intuitively, and don't forget to cleanse it every night after you have worn it.

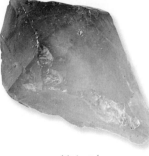

Natural amethyst

amethyst geode

AMETHYST

This is available as a geode (a hollow rock lined with crystals), a cluster or as single points that have been 'extracted' from another mineral.

Large geodes and clusters are good for placing in your healing space to maintain a high-frequency vibration, but remember always to keep them out of sunlight as they will fade in strong light.

Amethyst brings psychic gifts and is an excellent aid to meditation. However, it should not be used by anyone with mental disturbances such as schizophrenia, or with hyperactive children.

Violet light is known to reduce high blood pressure, reduce the appetite, calm shock and reconstruct the white blood corpuscles. Crystals of amethyst have a purifying, cleansing and antiseptic effect due to their colour, which verges into the ultraviolet range of higher and faster vibration. These crystals work directly on the Third Eye, the right brain (creative) area, the pineal gland and the pituitary gland. When we cooperate with amethyst, it opens our body to the energy of three newly emerging, transpersonal chakras above the head – the Causal Chakra, the Soul Star, and the Stellar Gateway. Crystal teachers are developing their understanding of these relatively new chakras.

CROWN CHAKRA MEDITATION

A good time for meditation is either following yoga practise or after crystal therapy. At such times, your body is already relaxed and ready for a session of focused concentration (see pages 22–23).

BEFORE YOU START

Choose a leisurely and relaxed time to meditate. If you like, create an atmosphere with oils, candles, or incense in the colour of the chakra. Sit or lie somewhere you won't be disturbed. You can pre-record the words of the meditation – dots indicate a pause.

1 As you sit or lie in your warm, silent, safe place, imagine a cap of a thousand white petals hugging the crown of your head.

2 Through the centre, where the petals meet, is an opening through which pours a golden/white/violet (choose) light ... This is your link with the Divine Source ... your connection with everything that ever was, is, or will be ...

3 Allow this light to pour in throughout your body ... nurturing every cell, every fibre of your being ... with pure consciousness ...

AFFIRMATIONS

- I tune into the union with my Higher Power.

- I am starting to accept myself as I am, with love and gratitude.

- I cease to limit myself intellectually and in my creativity and connect my spirit to the Source of all knowledge.

- I am a unique, radiant, loving being.

- I choose to transform my life and become free.

- I release all limited thoughts and lift myself up to ever higher levels of awareness.

- I am who I am.

4 A consciousness that transcends normal thought and the ordinary senses ... A consciousness taking you beyond space and time into a state of deeper awareness ...

5 This is your link with an unlimited realm of understanding, of knowing ...

6 Trust that everything in your life is unfolding exactly as it should, for your highest good ... Feel the power of this connection as the light bathes your body internally and externally with its Divine Radiance ...

7 You are now becoming enlightened ... the process of unlocking the mental blocks that have chained you to mundane realities in the past ...

8 Now you allow your mind to soar above its earthly shackles and detach itself from the limitations of your mortal mind ...

9 By doing so you are attaching yourself to your Higher Self ... to new experiences ... new beginnings ... a new awakening. Stay relaxed as you return to your normal surroundings.

DAILY QUESTIONS

- Do you retread familiar thought and behaviour patterns? Move into uncharted territory, available when you explore your Crown Chakra.

- Does your personal identification begin and end with job or economic status? List words describing the essential you. Add to the list daily.

- Can you reserve time for daily meditation? This is the key to achieving enlightenment.

- Are you in control of your destiny? Think back to when something wonderful happened. Did you control that event? Be open to coincidences that add magic to your life.

- Is there an issue in your life which you are battling to control through sheer willpower? Practice letting go of your desired outcome. Take a deep breath and tell yourself, 'I trust that the outcome will be for my highest good, no matter what it may be.' Then let go.

INDEX

ACKNOWLEDGEMENTS

Material previously published in
The Book of Chakra Healing (Gaia,
2013), and *The Chakra Bible* (Godsfield,
2007), divisions of Octopus Publishing
Group Ltd

Special Photography:
© **Octopus Publishing Group**/Ruth
Jenkinson

Other Photography:
akg-images/R. & S. Michaud 9; **Alamy**/
WoodyStock 143 bottom. **Corbis UK
Ltd** 29; /KG-Photography/zefa 27;
Octopus Publishing Group Ltd 38, 57,
59, 75, 76, 78, 71, 95, 96, 111, 113, 114, 115,
128, 129, 131, 133, 147, 148, 149, 151, 165,
167, 168, 169; /Colin Bowling 125 centre,
125 right, 143 t; /Stephen Conroy 125
left; /Frazer Cunningham 17, 19; /Ruth
Jenkinson 33, 34, 61; /Mike Prior 37,
39, 53; /Peter Pugh-Cook 107; /Russel
Sadur 23, 89, 112; /Ian Wallace 30.
Photodisc 97. **Thinkstock**/iStockphoto
20, 166. **TopFoto**/British Library Board/
Robana 2,45; /Charles Walker 11.

Illustrations: KJA Artists